FONTANUS MONOGRAPH SERIES
X

WESLEY BOURNE

THE QUINTESSENTIAL CANADIAN ANÆSTHETIST

The *Fontanus Monograph Series*
and the annual journal *Fontanus*,
published by the McGill University Libraries,
are devoted to the exploration
and presentation of the collections
of the McGill University libraries,
museums and archives.

General Editor: Hans Möller

X. Wesley Bourne, the Quintessential
Canadian Anæsthetist
1996.

175
1821 1996
McGill
MONTRÉAL

Joan C. Bevan, MD, FRCA

Research Anæsthetist, Brithish Columbia's Children's Hospital
and Associate Professor of Anæsthesia,
the University of British Columbia, Vancouver,
British Columbia, Canada

Maria A. Pacelli, BA

Administrative Coordinator, Department of Anesthesia,
McGill University, Montreal, Quebec, Canada

This book is dedicated to:

David R. Bevan, MB, MRCP, FRCA

Professor and Chairman, Department of Anæsthesia,
University of British Columbia, Vancouver,
British Columbia, Canada

and

First Wesley Bourne Professor in Anesthesia,
McGill University, Montreal, Quebec, Canada

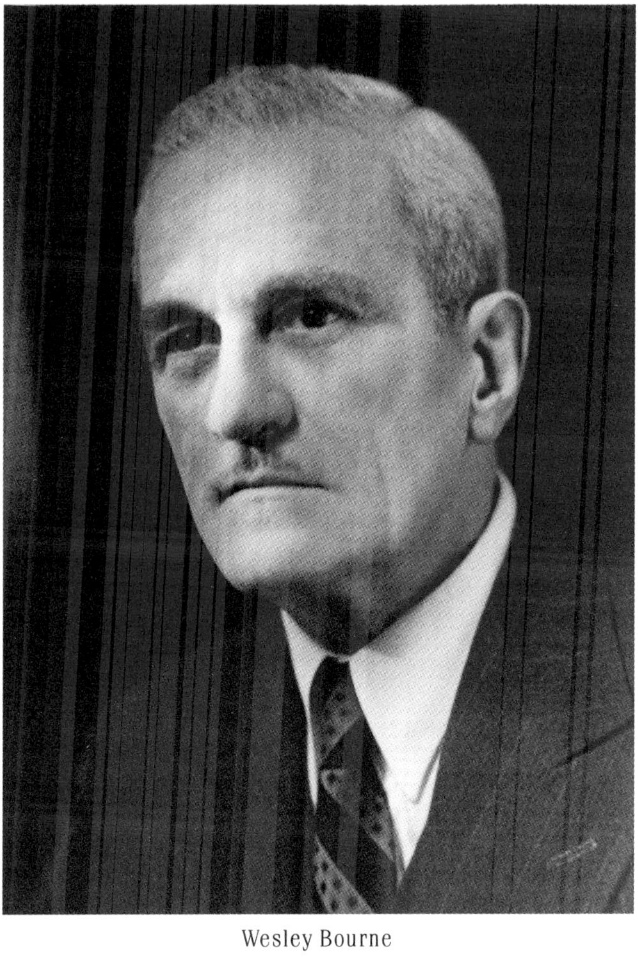

Wesley Bourne

FONTANUS MONOGRAPH SERIES
X

THE QUINTESSENTIAL CANADIAN ANÆSTHETIST

WESLEY BOURNE

A Retrospective on the Foundations of McGill Anesthesia

JOAN C. BEVAN
and
MARIA A. PACELLI

McGill University
Libraries
Montreal, 1996

General Editor: Hans Möller

Associate Editor: Lonnie Weatherby

Editorial Committee:
Martin Cohen, Peter Daly, Frances Groen,
John Hobbins, Pamela Miller, Hans Möller,
Richard Virr, Lonnie Weatherby

Word Processing: Elizabeth Thomson

Cover Design: Instructional Communications Centre, McGill

Printing: Les Editions Marquis Ltée

Paper: (∞) (acid-free) offset Mohawk Vellum

Published by the
McGill University Libraries
3459 McTavish Street
Montreal, PQ
H3A 1Y1

ISBN 0-7717-0485-2
ISSN 1183-1774

Contents

FOREWORD

The authors of this book, Joan Bevan and Maria Pacelli, have written a lively account of the life of Wesley Bourne. Originally from Barbados, Wesley Bourne spent his entire professional life, from medical student to emeritus professor, at McGill University in Montreal. Despite this, he was by no means parochial in outlook. He read widely, travelled extensively, and became an internationally-renowned leader in anæsthesia in the first half of the twentieth century. Each chapter provides a backdrop of life in the contemporary social, political and McGill University worlds. The work of other leading North American anæsthetists is mentioned, as is the impact of two world wars on life at McGill and on Wesley Bourne's career. His influence culminated in the establishment of the first academic department of anæsthesia in Canada with Wesley Bourne himself as its first chairman.

The authors vividly recount the various phases of Wesley Bourne's life, beginning with his childhood in Barbados. There, his early education led to a love of Greek and Latin classics from which he quoted extensively in his later writings. Having graduated MD McGill in 1911 and served as a captain in the RCAMC during the first world war, his energy and zest for life seemed unbounded and encompassed clinical work, pharmacological research, hobbies and family life. He raised the standard of clinical anæsthesia, pursued research in pharmacology, educated scores of students, developed an anæsthesia society in Montreal and joined national and international societies to exchange information and raise the profile of anæsthesia. The authors have captured the essence of Wesley Bourne's contributions which always had what Harold Griffith described as "the flame of passionate idealism." The authors have achieved a balance between Wesley Bourne's own contributions and those that he made jointly with his contemporaries at McGill and in the wider world of anæsthesia.

Fifty years later, as the second half of the twentieth century draws to a close, anæsthetists take for granted the need for research and organized teaching, professional organizations and scientific meetings. In all of these developments, Wesley Bourne played an influential role. His honours were many, including election as President of both the International Anesthesia Research Society and the American Society of Anesthesiologists in the United States, and the receipt of the Henry Hill Hickman medal of the Royal Society in England. His three-year McGill Diploma Course in Anæsthesia became a model for specialist anæsthetic training throughout Canada. But perhaps his most important achievement was that, through his contributions, others recognized that anæsthesia was an academic medical specialty that deserved equal recognition with all others.

By describing the life of Wesley Bourne in the context of the founding and development of the McGill Department of Anesthesia in Montreal, the authors give perspective to the growth of organized anæsthetic and academic departments in twentieth century North America. Readers of the book will feel the excitement of knowing a great man who was part of these achievements.

J.R. Maltby
Professor of Anæsthesia
Foothills Hospital and the
University of Calgary
Calgary, Alberta

PREFACE

To write a biography of Wesley Bourne is to also comprehend the history of the McGill Department of Anæsthesia. His family history, professional role, achievements and contributions to anæsthesia will be examined in the context of the development of medical knowledge at the time, and the cirucumstances and events influencing Dr. Bourne's career will be recounted. The source of much of the material is in Dr. Bourne's own published articles. These have been quoted liberally to reveal the nature of his thinking. The stimulus for further research came from reading an address given by one of his successors to the Chair, Dr. Richard R.G. Gilbert, who delivered "A Tribute to Wesley Bourne" as the 1977 Wesley Bourne Memorial Lecturer. Throughout, the Bourne family encouraged and supported this effort: Dr. Bourne's sons, Mr. J. Douglas Bourne, Mr. John G. Bourne and Dr. Robert H. Bourne, provided anecdotes of home life. Douglas, assisted by Dr. Jamie Bourne (Hilary's son), researched the family tree. With the support of a library fellowship, Maria Pacelli visited the Wood Library Museum of the American Society of Anesthesiologists in Chicago. Much of Dr. Bourne's memorabilia was housed in the library after his death, and Maria received invaluable assistance from the librarian, Patrick Sims, in locating this material. Of all those who helped in the quest for the title and author of the poem *The Bridge Builder,* credit is due to Ms. Donna MacFarlane, the McGill residency programme secretary, who was successful after a very long search.

Amongst present faculty members, Dr. John Sandison provided his copy of *Mysterious Waters to Guard,* Dr. Deirdre Gillies shared her recollections of Dr. Bourne, whom she had known since her childhood and Dr. Gordon S. Fox, a member of the Quarter Century Club after serving for twenty-five years on the McGill faculty, supplied historical medical journals. Dr. Jean-Pierre Tétreault, Université de Sherbrooke, Québec, found records left by his uncle, Dr. Georges Cousineau, of meetings between English and French anæsthetists in Montreal. Ms. Ann Wright transcribed text of the Wesley Bourne Memorial Lectures, which were available on audiotapes from 1974, and Chantal Villemure helped to compile the list of publications.

Joan Bevan delved in the historical archives of the Health Sciences Library at McGill, a treasure trove of medical texts and journals spanning the last century and also home to the Osler Library of the History of Medicine. Almost complete sets of the first anæsthesia journals were shelved in the basement. *The Quarterly Anesthesia Supplement of the American Journal of Surgery,* from its first issue in October 1914 until it was superceded by a separate publication, *Current Researches in Anesthesia and Analgesia* in August 1922, are held by the library. This title later became *Anesthesia and Analgesia, Current Researches* in 1957 and has been known as *Anesthesia and Analgesia* since 1979. The *Canadian Medical Association Journal* began in 1911 and provided a forum for publications in all specialties. The second anæsthesia journal, the *British Journal of Anæsthesia*, appeared just one year after the first, in 1923 and was joined by *Anæsthesia* in 1946. The *Canadian Anæsthetists' Society Journal* began publication in 1954 and the name was changed to the *Canadian Journal of Anæsthesia/Journal Canadien d'Anesthésie* in 1987. These journals provided insights into the state of medicine and the development of anæsthesia in Canada in those early years, and were invaluable in tracing the history of Canadian anæsthesia, and placing Wesley Bourne in the context of his time.

During the course of these researches, three books were published which amplified knowledge of the history surrounding Wesley Bourne and McGill and served to bring together so many of the fragments of this story. In 1992, "Harold Griffith," by Drs. Richard Bodman and Deirdre Gillies[1], and *Harold Griffith: His Life and Legacy* edited by Drs. J. Roger Maltby and David A.E. Shephard[2] were published, and were followed in 1993 by *Watching Closely Those Who Sleep: A History of the Canadian Anæsthetists' Society* by Dr. David A.E. Shephard[3]. In combination with the 1980 and 1984 volumes of *McGill University for the Advancement of Learning* by Stanley Brice Frost[4], detailing the University's history and development, these sources describe the contemporaneous professional and societal relationships which existed in Canada. International links were documented in *Fifty years: The Australian Society of Anæsthetists* by Gwen Wilson[5] and *Five Decades: The South African Society of Anæsthetists* by Nagin Parbhoo[6] published in 1987 and 1993, respectively. Thus, a burden of uncertainty about the prevailing circumstances of Wesley Bourne's professional life was removed, and it became easier to write this biographical account of the founding chairman of McGill Anæsthesia.

Notwithstanding the inevitable omissions, which may generate controversy and expose the inevitable tensions, arguments and conflicts inherent in a successful careeer, this has been a satisfying undertaking. At times the truth seemed elusive, and the facts would not coalesce into a meaningful whole but these were only temporary reverses. The spur was always there to promote an awareness of Wesley Bourne, a remarkable man whose legacy permeates the past, present and future of McGill Anæsthesia.

Preface

In his obituary for the *Canadian Anæsthetists' Society Journal* (1965), Dr. Harold R. Griffith praised him with these words:

> A light which for more than fifty years has illuminated the whole field of anæsthesiology has flickered and gone out.......To countless anæsthesiologists throughout the world he has been an inspiration, a stimulus, a teacher, and a great friend.[7] (*Can Anaesth Soc J* 1965, 12:315-17)

References

1. Bodman, R. and D. Gillies. "Harold Griffith. The evolution of modern anæsthesia." In: Morley T.P. (Series Ed). *Canadian Medical Lives*, no. 8. Toronto, Oxford: Hannah Institute and Dundurn Press, 1992.
2. Maltby, J.R. and D.A.E. Shephard (Eds.). "Harold Griffith. His life and legacy: a tribute on the 50th anniversary of the introduction of curare into anæsthetic practice." Published by the Canadian Anæsthetists' Society as a supplement to *Canadian Journal of Anæsthesia* 1992;39 no.1 (Jan).
3. Shephard, D.A.E. "Watching Closely Those Who Sleep. A history of the Canadian Anæsthetists' Society 1943-93." Published by the Canadian Anæsthetists' Society as a supplement to *Canandian Journal of Anæsthesia* 1993;40 no.6 (June).
4. Frost, S.B. *McGill University: for the Advancement of Learning*, vol. 1, 1801-95 and vol. 2, 1895-1971. Kingston, Montreal: McGill-Queen's University Press, 1980 and 1984.
5. Wilson G. *Fifty Years. The Australian Society of Anæsthetists 1934-84.* Australian Society of Anæsthetists, 1987.
6. Parbhoo N. *Five Decades. The South African Society of Anæsthetists 1943-93*. South African Society of Anæsthetists, 1993.
7. Griffith, Harold R.

I

Growing Up In Barbados (1886-1907)

One thing was clear from the beginning: Wesley Bourne was going to be successful. He had a capacity for work and an overwhelming enjoyment of life, with an intense perception of his environment. However, in his youth in Barbados, it is unlikely that he imagined himself as one of the pioneers in the emerging specialty of anæsthesia, or as pivotal to the establishment and development of the McGill Department of Anesthesia. Nevertheless, those were the achievements of a career which spanned two world wars and saw medicine advance at an unprecedented pace. Each phase of his life, from his birth on 24th April, 1886 in St. Philip, Barbados, to his death in his 79th year on 26th February, 1965 in Montreal, provides insight into the moulding of this special man.

The family boasts a colourful ancestry. Wesley Bourne claimed English descent from a Somerset family whose three brothers took part in the 1685 rebellion against the Duke of Monmouth. They were captured, tried and "Barbadosed" by Judge Jeffreys. One was deported to St. Vincent, one to the Carolinas and one to Barbados. The veracity of this account could not be confirmed by a genealogical search in Barbados. The search identified Thomas Bourne (1798-1846), a shoemaker, heading the family tree. Next came Henry, grandfather of Wesley Bourne, recorded as a plumber; but actually believed to be a cooper, who made the barrels used to boil down sugar to make molasses. Another line began with a John Bourne, who was sent to Barbados as an indentured servant, or slave, and died in 1684, just before the Monmouth uprising. This line terminated with another Thomas Bourne, who could only have been seventeen years old when Thomas, the shoemaker, who was not related, was born.

Barbadians are the descendants of only a few early English colonists and their West African slaves, whom they imported to labour on the plantations. There was little foreign immigration. The island remained under British rule for three centuries before attaining independence as a Commonwealth state in 1966. The uprising of 1865 had been quelled, but racial intolerance remained a feature of Barbados' culture in Wesley Bourne's youth. Blacks always outnumbered the whites and now make up about ninety percent of the population. Among the 15,000 whites now living on the island, there are still a number of "red legs," the slang designation for the released indentured servants and their descendants. After they were freed, they were compelled to live a very primitive existence, and some remain in that state to this day. It is possible that family records have been lost or may have been destroyed by hurricane or fire. Therefore, if Wesley Bourne's version of his ancestry is true, it is unlikely that it will ever be verified.

Wesley Bourne was born on a sugar cane plantation, owned and operated by his father. It was known as "Pollards," and was located in the parish of St. Philip, Barbados. He was the fourth of five children of James Thomas Bourne (1851-1923) and Mary Elizabeth Harding (1849-1937). He had three brothers and one sister. His father, usually known as Tom, so loved the hymns of Charles Wesley (1707-88) that he gave the name "Wesley" to his son. An interesting anecdote is related regarding his decision to baptize his children giving them only one name. He argued that he had been given two names, but used only one of them and, besides, it was less difficult to choose only one name. When Wesley registered at McGill he was asked his name and replied "Wesley." The next question was "What is your other name?" To this, Wesley responded "I don't have one." This elicited "Oh, but you must have two names." Whereupon he chose as his middle name "Luke," which was a spur of the moment decision that reflected his deep religious convictions at that time (in fact, the Bishop of Barbados tried hard to entice Wesley into entering the priesthood, but he stood his ground and enrolled at McGill). Knowing that St. Luke had been a physician before becoming an apostle of Jesus, probably prompted his choice.

Tom Bourne, by all accounts, led a full and gregarious life, despite the financial vagaries associated with the life of a Barbadian planter. He was musical, with a good singing voice and taught himself to play the piano and violin. He loved to organize a dance, sometimes at short notice, to the discomfiture of his wife, Mamie. Pauline, their granddaughter, recalls that her mother, Blanche, Wesley's sister, talked about watching Tom and Mamie dance together, with Mamie wearing a red rose.

Although involved in charismatic evangelism and a local leader for visits to neighbouring parishes, Tom was also fond of shooting parties and had a reputation for being the best shot on the island. When it was his turn to be host, the officers of the garrison loved to vie with him and good food and drink were plentiful. His sense of correctness was evident. One of Wesley's fondest memories, passed on to his own children was, when he was of age, of being taken in his buggy to his club for his first drink. He came to realize that Tom was generous towards his family and friends when they found themselves in financial need. Wesley's parents spent their retirement years together at "Newhaven" in Foul Bay, on the southern shore of the island until his father's death, supposedly as a result of poor medical care, in 1923 at the age of seventy two. Douglas Bourne, Wesley's son, recalls visiting Mamie, who was living with his cousin Alan[1], in 1931. The house was surrounded by a balcony with steps that led down to the beach. Douglas still wonders whether Tom kept the custom, during his final years, of going down to bathe in the sea, as he had seen some elderly white gentlemen do at Worthing beach, on the south coast of England, recently.

All of Tom Bourne's five children became successful: Wesley's story is familiar, two of his brothers became ordained priests, one did well as a plantation owner and manager, and his sister was an able and respected school teacher. James Bourne (1878-1935), Wesley's brother and his senior by only eight years, had considerable influence on his early years and later life. He was godfather to his nephew, Wesley's son Douglas, who remembers him as, "Uncle Jimmie." He had graduated from Bishop's College, Lennoxville, Quebec and studied theology in Philadelphia, qualifying for the Anglican ministry and the Episcopalian Church, into which he had been ordained in 1902. Dissatisfaction with this church soon caused him to join with a classmate, Edward Hawkes, in leading thirty or more similarly disposed clergymen into the Roman Catholic Church, (as recounted in a book by Father Hawkes) and in 1906 he was ordained into the Roman Catholic Church. He was the founder and first pastor of St. Rose of Lima Church in Philadelphia, where he oversaw the construction of a new presbytery for the parish, which still stands today. He enjoyed a full life, having the service of a car with chauffeur-valet, playing golf and socializing with prominent parishoners.

There was a close family relationship. James travelled to Montreal for holidays, including at least one fishing trip at the Winchester Club, in the Laurentian hills, northeast of Montreal. On one visit to Barbados, Wesley composed the parody "Bye, Bye, Barbados" based on "Bye, Bye Blackbird," which went something like this: "Put your troubles to the bar, Here we come,

---

[1] Cousin Alan was one of the family members who had been helped financially by Wesley Bourne's father, Tom. Mamie was living with him at the time of Douglas' visit. Alan was a pharmacist and his grandson continues to operate the retail business, which has prospered, and has expanded into manufacturing in Barbados and wholesaling throughout the islands.

full of rum, Bye, bye Barbados." James had a great interest in literature and art and gave the children gifts of two beautiful volumes of reproduction paintings and a complete set of the works of Charles Dickens. Douglas still has a copy of Balthazar Gracian's *The Art of Worldly Wisdom*, with a note on the inside cover "Douglas, for your pocket, Uncle Jimmie," as well as hand-painted mounted miniatures of his uncle and his grandmother, Mamie. James Bourne suffered from diabetes and poor health forced him to accept less onerous duties in 1928. For a time, he was rector at a new convent associated with the parish of St. Joan of Arc in Philadelphia, where his life-long friend, Monsignor Edward Hawkes was pastor. At the time of his death, seven years later, he was chaplain of Philadelphia's Catholic Home for Destitute Children.

Wesley Bourne received his primary education at Lodge school, located about four miles from his home in the adjoining parish of St. John. His education under his headmaster, an Oxonian scholar and teacher of the classics, was approached with his characteristic total dedication. His broadened horizons, were helped in some measure by the assistance of two very salutary canings, according to Dr. Harold Griffith[2], later his closest associate in Montreal[3]. The school provided an excellent grounding in English, Latin, Greek, mathematics, chemistry, religious studies and botany. These early studies imbued him with a love of books and the Greek and Latin which embellished much of his later writing; while the indelible, guiding principles learned in his childhood home amongst this devout family would remain throughout his life. Wesley Bourne was happy on the tropical plantation, with proximity to open country and ocean, but his active, inquisitive and retentive mind was stimulated and he was enthusiastic about continuing his education. His decision to study medicine was probably taken on the advice of his headmaster, Mr. Emptage and McGill was the university of choice for many Barbadians at that time[4].

---

[2] Griffith, H.R. "Eminent anæsthetists, no. 6: Wesley Bourne." *British Journal of Anæsthesia* 1951;23:186-95.

[3] To many, it appeared that Harold Griffith was Wesley Bourne's closest friend, as well as his associate in Montreal. However, James Douglas Bourne says that Colonel A.H. Cowie was probably his father's closest friend, despite the strong professional relationship between Griffith and Bourne.

[4] Dr. R.G.B. Gilbert, and others who wrote tributes to Wesley Bourne, could not explain Wesley Bourne's reasons for coming to McGill University to study medicine. To Wesley's eldest son, James Douglas, it was quite obvious that McGill was simply the first choice for Barbadians, and it was gaining an international reputation. He knew of no family connections in Montreal, but Wesley's older brother, James, had graduated from nearby Bishops' University in Lennoxville, Quebec.

Wesley Bourne must have been aware that much of medicine in the late nineteenth and early twentieth centuries was influenced by the great Canadian physician, Sir William Osler (1849-1919)[5]. In 1870, Osler moved from Toronto to Montreal, at the same time his teacher, Dr. James Bovell, on whose mentorship he relied during his schooling at Weston school in Ontario, went to the West Indies. Osler graduated from McGill in 1872 and went on to work in the wards of Montreal General Hospital; always stressing the importance of laboratory work and research, while establishing his reputation and founding medical societies. After fourteen years in Montreal, one year before Wesley's birth, Osler moved to Philadelphia. His impact, as the most renowned physician of his day, was still evident in Montreal. The challenges in medicine were enormous and anæsthesia was in its infancy. The medical journals of the day provided examples of contemporary clinical practice and the limits of anæsthetic practice at the turn of the century. Nitrous oxide and ether were the most commonly used agents[6] and chloroform was linked to deaths under anæsthesia[7]. It was not unusual for surgery to be performed with little or no anæsthesia[8].

In 1907 Wesley Bourne left Barbados for Montreal to enrol in the McGill University Faculty of Medicine. He knew that his father hoped that he would return to Barbados to practice medicine, but this was not to be.

---

[5] Noble, I. *The Doctor Who Dared. William Osler.* Vancouver, Toronto, Montreal: The Copp Clark Publishing Co, Ltd., 1959.

[6] "Nitrous oxide and ether anæsthesia, the nitrous oxide being used as a preliminary to ether, has been employed in England for a good many years, but until recently has been little used in this country." (Carter, H.W. "Nitrous oxide and ether anæsthesia." *Medical Record*, New York. 14 April 1900:627.)

[7] "The second case was that of a man aged forty-seven years, the subject of chronic hip disease for forty-three years. He died during chloroform anæsthesia." (Cornell, S.S. "Clinical notes." Abstract from *The Montreal Medical Journal*, February, 1900. *Medical Record*, New York. 14 April 1900:647.)

[8] "Jasper Cargill reports this case, in which his patient, a black woman in Jamaica, while suffering the removal of a leg under chloroform, showed symptoms of heart failure. When told that the operation could not go on, she said: "Please cut it off, doctor; I can stand it without chloroform." After a brief consultation this was accordingly done, without a sign of resistance or even a groan from the patient." (Cargill, J. "Amputation without anæsthesia." Abstract from *British Medical Journal*, 31 March, 1900. *Medical Record*, New York. 14 April 1900:643).

II

EARLY MCGILL YEARS (1907-18)

When Wesley Bourne entered McGill in 1907, Montreal had a population of 300,000, almost evenly divided between people of English and French origin. The city was developing as a commercial centre and was the birthplace of a number of his future colleagues, including Drs. Harold R. Griffith (1894-1985) and Georges Cousineau (1906-1987). It was also home to some interesting personalities like the widowed Mrs. Anna Leonowens, better known as "Anna of Siam" from her days as governess to the King's children in that country. She lived in the Square Mile, close to the University near the top of McTavish, from 1891 until her death at eighty-four years of age in 1915. During that time she devoted herself to philanthropic, religious and charitable works for the community. Her service as president of the Montreal Foundling and Baby Hospital is commemorated on a plaque which now hangs in Montreal Children's Hospital. At her funeral service, held in Christ Church Cathedral on St Catherine Street, Professor John Macnaughton of the classics department at McGill paid tribute to her as the best, bravest and wisest of all women he had met.

Wesley Bourne arrived on a much more rural campus than exists today. A granite monument in the centre of the lower campus marked the burial spot of the remains of James McGill, the founder of the University. In 1875, they had been moved from a cemetery on Dorchester Boulevard and it is believed that some of the bones of his friend and business partner, John Porteus, were mistakenly buried alongside those of McGill. James McGill was thought to have planted an elm tree, a campus landmark, about 1790. A catastrophic fire, in the year of Wesley Bourne's arrival, destroyed most of the University's medical building and forced the faculty into temporary quarters until the Strathcona Building, built near the Royal Victoria Hospital, was opened in 1911. The student body at McGill was fairly homogeneous, composed of less than 2,500 men and women who were mostly English-speaking Protestants from middle-class backgrounds, despite the rapidly increasing proportion of the French population and immigrant migration from other countries to Montreal and the surrounding areas.

There were two French medical schools in Montreal; L'École de Médecine et de Chirurgie de Montréal (which could not grant degrees, depriving its graduates of licences to practice medicine in Quebec), and the medical school affiliated with the medical faculty of Laval University. These joined to form the medical faculty of the Université de Montréal in 1919. Women were not admitted to the McGill medical program before World War I. The first women graduated in 1922. However, Maude Abbott (1869-1940), who was among the women who graduated from the medical faculty of Bishop's University at Lennoxville, Quebec, was acknowledged a McGill graduate when the medical faculties merged in 1905.

Sir Thomas Roddick (1846-1923), surgeon-in-chief at the Royal Victoria Hospital, was Dean of Medicine until 1908. He had organized medical services in the field during the Riel Rebellion, but his greatest achievements were in medical politics. He negotiated the agreement which brought the McGill Faculty of Medicine under University administration in 1905, and was the author of the Canada Medical Act which received royal assent in 1906. It took another five years before all nine provinces agreed, but an amended act was passed in 1911 and the Medical Council of Canada was established. This meant that holders of the diploma from the Council had the right to practice medicine anywhere in Canada. The diploma also provided medical reciprocity with Britain, and a practitioner could serve in the medical services of the Army and Navy.

The Faculty of Medicine had been established since 1822 and was recognized for the strength of its clinical teaching embodying the principles of medical research and enquiry propounded by Sir William Osler. In this tradition, medical science and clinical practice were closely allied, so that it was easy for clinicians to work in hospital laboratories; and researchers and lecturers made no distinction between their scientific and clinical teaching roles, regardless of whether their funding sources originated with the University or hospital. Wesley Bourne was taught medicine by Osler's pupils—Francis Shepherd, Dean of Medicine and J. George Adami, professor of pathology. He achieved first place in anatomy and graduated in 1911 as conjoint Doctor of Medicine and Master of Surgery (MD CM). When he had obtained his degree, he asked the university principal, Dean William Peterson, an Edinburgh and Oxford scholar, what he thought about practicing medicine in Montreal. The Dean replied, "Well, Bourne, the first thing you will have to do is to get rid of that dreadful Barbadian accent."He would later tell that story against himself, but he did lose the accent although it would sometimes re-emerge when agitated.

The fluctuating fortunes of the sugar industry in Barbados, compelled Wesley Bourne to find work quickly. Doctors were badly needed to look after the construction workers on the Canadian Pacific Railway in Alberta[1]. The working environment was hazardous and many were injured. The unsanitary conditions in the construction camps caused the spread of infections by insects and the contamination of water. Thousands were migrating to find work and villages were growing up around the railway. The only doctors available were recent medical graduates from the medical school in Manitoba or from the East[2]. Some of these railroad doctors stayed on as community practitioners in the settlements, but Wesley Bourne worked there only for a year in order to earn sufficient money to return to Montreal in 1913, to train in surgery at the Royal Victoria Hospital with Edward Archibald[3], a brilliant thoracic surgeon interested in pulmonary tuberculosis.

Infectious diseases, tuberculosis, syphilis and osteomyelitis were endemic and treatment was directed towards asepsis and antisepsis in surgery. These fundamental principles had been postulated by Joseph Lord Lister (1827-1912). Sir Thomas Roddick had accepted Lister's germ theories (first introduced into surgical practice in 1877) and thousands of lives were being saved simply by keeping wounds clean using antisepsis with carbolic acid and iodine as a disinfectant, or by nursing tuberculous patients outdoors in the fresh air of a country sanitorium. Diagnostic X-rays had been introduced in early 1896, and the correlation between skin exposure and cancer, or sterility after radiation of the ovaries and testes, was recognized in the first decade of use, leading to the use of protective measures. Anæsthesia depended on the use of local anæsthetics, spinal anæsthesia, chloroform, ether, nitrous oxide and ethyl chloride, with general anæsthesia used in essential surgery, tonsil removal, excision of tumours, or dental extractions.

---

[1] The Canadian Pacific Railway (CPR) was incorporated in 1881 and arrived in Calgary in 1883. The Calgary to Edmonton line was completed in 1891 and the last spike was driven in 1885 at Eagle Pass in British Columbia. Between 1917 and 1923 the Government of Canada formed the Canadian National Railway (CNR), which was in competition with the CPR, but both survived. In 1912, Wesley Bourne may have worked in the West for CPR but the exact location is not known (although the railroad appears to have been completed earlier). He could not have worked for CNR. Tributes by Dr. Harold Griffith and Dr. Dick Gilbert were the source of this information. Mr. John Bourne thinks his father actually worked on railroad construction in Northern Ontario, not in the West. This would explain the lack of correlation with CPR and CNR records.

[2] Bruner, M. "Early Medicine in Alberta." *Doctor's Review*, February 1987, 86-9 & 105.

[3] Dr. Edward Archibald was interested in teaching and encouraging young doctors. Dr. Norman Bethune worked under him from 1928-1932, during which time Bethune developed the rib shears which became popular for chest surgery.

The use of plasma for blood replacement, and the recognition that ventricular fibrillation precipitated deaths under chloroform, were now medical advances that went beyond the common practices of giving open drop ether and chloroform.

Great debates were looming about whether general anæsthesia should be administered by physicians or non-physicians and what sort of training in anæsthesia, if any, was needed. Comparisons of morbidity and mortality were drawn between untrained interns and their trained anæsthetist counterparts. The interns used three times more ether, administered stimulants to six times as many patients and produced almost twice as much post-operative vomiting for longer periods[4]. Some surgeons recommended that anæsthesia should be placed in trained, professional hands and that the anæsthetist should be accepted as a member of the surgical team[5]. Others pushed for legalization of the status of nurses who administered anæsthetics. They expressed views such as:

> "If practically their employment has been advantageous to the surgical service without in the slightest degree endangering the patients, it is difficult to maintain that nurses with a lack of medical training cannot be efficient anesthetists" or "Do surgeons desire nurses to administer anesthetics? If the answer is in the affirmative, the laws should be altered so as to include the administration of anesthetics within the activities delegated to the nursing profession. If surgeons are opposed to nurse anesthetists, no legislation is necessary. It merely remains for the profession to discontinue the use of nurse in this capacity and to discourage their employment in hospitals, private institutions and private practice."[6]

However, there was a growing sense that anæsthesia needed to be a medical sub-specialty. Dr. Frank McMechan (1879-1939) of Cincinnatti, Ohio, whose clinical practice was cut short in 1915 by crippling arthritis, used his organizational genius to establish anæsthesia societies and publish the first journal in anæsthesia, as a means of promoting the notion that the technique of

---

[4] Williams, E. "Anesthesisa by untrained anesthetists." *American Journal of Surgery* 1911;25:360. (Abstract from *St. Louis Medical Review*).

[5] Bevan, A.D. "Conclusions concerning anesthetics." *American Journal of Surgery* 1913;27:392. (Abstract from *Surgery Gynecology and Obstetrics.*)

[6] "Nurses as anæsthetists." [Editorial]. *American Journal of Surgery* 1914; 28:321-2.

administering anæsthetics should be the prerogative of physicians. His journal started in 1914 as the *Quarterly Supplement of Anesthesia and Analgesia* in the *American Journal of Surgery*, later became an independent journal, *Current Researches in Anesthesia and Analgesia*, in 1922. The introductory number of the *Quarterly Supplement* included a paper on insufflation anæsthesia by Dr. F.W. Nagle of the Royal Victoria Hospital, Montreal.[7] In the same issue, post-operative nausea and vomiting, spinal anæsthesia and local anæsthesia for herniorrhaphy were discussed.

This journal filled the need to communicate the theory and practice of anæsthesia and to exchange political views among members of the budding societies interested in anæsthesia as a speciality. In 1893, Dr. Frederick Silk had founded the Society of Anæsthetists in London, England and this became the Section of Anæsthetics of the Royal Society of Medicine in 1908. In North America the first society of anæsthetists, the Long Island Society of Anesthetists was founded in 1905 and evolved into the American Society of Anesthesiologists in 1944. In 1911 it existed as the New York Society of Anesthetists, but was not a national body. Dr. Frank McMechan envisaged a large society formed by the amalgamation of regional groups, and in 1912 he founded the American Association of Anesthetists which embraced the Scottish Society of Anesthetists, the Interstate Association of Anesthetists, New York Society of Anesthetists, followed by the Providence (RI) Society of Anesthetists in 1916. Another publication, the *American Year Book of Anesthesia and Analgesia*, was advertised for sale at $4. The first volume was for 1915-16.

Attention was focussed on the design of an apparatus for the more precise delivery of anæsthetic gases. One example, the Alcock chloroform vaporizer, a calibrated temperature-compensated plenum apparatus was described in 1908. This vaporizer had the advantage of portability, particularly appropriate to the itinerant anæsthestist. Its inventor, Dr. Nathaniel Henry Alcock, held the chair of physiology at McGill for two years until his death from leukæmia in 1913.

When Wesley Bourne began his surgical training, few physicians practiced anæsthesia full-time and there were no designated teaching departments

---

[7] Nagle, F.W. "Insufflation anesthesia." *Quarterly Supplement of Anesthesia and Analgesia. American Journal of Surgery* 1914;28:17-8.

for anæsthesia. Dr. Francis Willard Nagle (1880-1918), chief anæsthetist and lecturer in anæsthetics as well as a demonstrator in pharmacology, was the sole anæsthetist at the Royal Victoria Hospital and he needed assistance. He asked Wesley Bourne to try his hand at dropping ether. Presumably, Bourne's financial difficulties had not been alleviated and he considered administering anæsthetics for a while as a means of earning his living. However, he found it so fascinating that he decided to make it his profession. Dr. Nagle was an advocate of endotracheal anæsthesia and, under his tutelage, Bourne was introduced to anæsthesia and gradually developed his clinical skills. His decision to practice anæsthesia coincided with another pivotal event in his life: he married Sara Beatrice McGillis, of Montreal, on Wednesday, 29th November, 1913. They had four children, James Douglas, John Gilbert, Barbara Jean and Robert Henry.

The more widespread use of anæsthesia on relatively healthy patients prompted an examination of the mortality associated with anæsthesia. Blame was apportioned to both the anæsthetist and to the anæsthetic agents. Medico-legal cases concerning deaths under anæsthesia administered by non-medical anæsthetists began to be reported in the *Quarterly Anesthesia Supplement*. In 1915, the case of *Nations vs. Ludington, Wells and Van Schaik Lumber Co.* (concerning a labourer who died under anæsthesia, before surgery started) in Louisiana, resulted in the awarding of $10,000 in damages and a directive from the Supreme Court that only a physician should have been employed to give the anæsthetic[8].On the other hand, a similar case in the District of Columbia, *Levy vs. Vaughan*, found that a medical student administering ether to a high risk patient had no liability in the patient's death[9].

The first mention that anæsthetic records could be helpful in assessing the work of anæsthetists appeared in the *Quarterly Anesthesia Supplement* in 1916 accompanied by reports of mortality rates of 1 in 14,000 for all general anæsthetics, with an increase to 1 in 2,000 when chloroform was used. This

---

[8] "Medico-legal aspects of anesthesia and analgesia. Liability of employer for death of employee under operation, when layman administers the anæsthetic" *Quarterly Supplement of Anesthesia and Analgesia. American Journal of Surgery* 1915;29:60. (Abstract from the *Medical Record*, February 28, 1914).

[9] "Medico-legal aspects of anesthesia and analgesia. Surgeon not liable for death due to anesthetic administered by medical student." *Quarterly Supplement of Anesthesia and Analgesia. American Journal of Surgery* 1915;29:59.

suggested that it would have been comparatively safer to use ether and nitrous oxide, the other commonly-used agents at the time. Statistics of over two million cases were compiled from reliable sources and were published, indicating decreased mortality and demonstrating the relative safety of different agents: deaths from ether were 1 in 8,010; chloroform, 1 in 2,605; ethyl chloride, 1 in 13,365; spinal anæsthesia, 1 in 515; scopolamine, 1 in 666. The Committee on Anesthesia of the American Medical Association interpreted this as a constraint on the use of chloroform except as an induction agent before ether, and the American Association of Anesthetists proposed the mandatory collection of mortality statistics employing a standardized anæsthetic chart. These views stimulated considerable correspondence concerning the difficulties inherent in collecting accurate statistics from private and hospital practitioners and indicated that a hospital-record keeping system would be the most appropriate method.

However, these arguments were coloured by the continuing battle between physician-anæsthetists, who wanted to eliminate non-physician anæsthesia altogether, and surgeons and hospital administrators who saw the convenience and cheapness of non-physicians. Dr. F.D. Bullard's address to the third annual meeting of the American Association of Anæsthetists included some resonant comments:

> The ideal anesthetist should be well informed, confident, tactful, observing, judicial, quick to act, watchful and cool. I believe also he or she should have a full medical training. Such a person who has developed an aptness for this dangerous and absolutely essential work should be treated by the surgeon, the profession, and the laity in an appropriate manner. Professional honors and adequate financial recompense should be his reward.

The number of physician anæsthetists, full or part time, was too small to cope with the increasing demands for clinical service. In Montreal, administrators swelled the ranks by recruiting interns from around the hospital and had them work on an apprenticeship system. This was apparently no worse than elsewhere in North America. Dr. Willis D. Gatch, professor of surgery at the University of Indiana, Indianapolis, in his presidential address to the fourth annual meeting of the American Association of Anesthetists in 1916, outlined his goals for training students in anæsthesia describing his own practice of making all medical students perform at least ten anæsthetics under the supervision of a trained anæsthetist. He subsequently drew attention to the woeful inadequacies of anæsthesia training:

> Unless our medical schools give instruction in anesthesia not described in their catalogues, the training of students in this subject must be either entirely lacking or very inadequate. Such personal inquiries as I have been able to make of medical teachers convinces me that this is the case.

In the United States, Georgia, Kentucky, Ohio, Michigan and later West Virginia, Indiana and Tennessee, aligned themselves with the Interstate Association of Anesthetists in limiting the administration of anæsthesia to licensed physicians by 1917. Dr. J.M. Baldy, president of the Bureau of Medical Education and Licensure in Pennsylvania wrote to Dr. F. McMechan:

> The condition of the administration of anesthesia and the pitiable dependency of the patient upon utterly incompetent doctors, is depicted in that address. It holds absolutely good today, and so far as I can see, as a medical man, the future is as dark as the past; at any rate within the limits of our lifetime. If your society could provide a sufficiency of competent anesthetists for this country, no one would hail the fact with greater glee than would I. But you, as a body, are not a grain of sand in fulfilling that want. If I could see the possibility of the medical hospitals of the country being able to financially employ a medical man for full-time service (that is full-time as applied to their individual requirements), both for the giving of anesthesia and the teaching of the interne, I would be inclined to adopt your position.

During this time, McGill was preparing for war and Wesley Bourne served as a captain in the local army unit. The Canadian Officers' Training Corps was established at McGill in 1912; the first in any Canadian university. As soon as war was declared, the Graduates' Society began to organize the McGill Provisional Battalion, a volunteer training unit which supplied many recruits for the regular Canadian forces. These two units soon combined to form the nucleus of the Canadian Universities Company of Light Infantry. Later, one tank and two artillery battalions were formed. Over 3,000 McGill graduates and students, at least sixty percent of eligible men, were recruited for combat. The medical faculty played a major part in the war effort. Dr. John McCrae (1872-1918), a pathologist from the Royal Victoria Hospital created the poem

"In Flander's Fields." Osler, by now in his sixties, was an honorary colonel who worked tirelessly not only for the Canadian Hospital in London and the Canadian Military Hospital, Folkestone, England but also for the War Relief Fund. His son, Revere, who was an orderly officer in the McGill unit and later a lieutenant, lost his life in shell fire in Flanders. He was tended by Dr. Harvey Cushing.

World War I caused numerous changes in anæsthesiology. The brutality of war and the suffering of its victims spurred medical science to find improved methods to alleviate pain. It is worth re-reading some of the accounts of wartime experiences; that of Dr. William Boyman Howell[10] of Montreal which he presented to the sixth meeting of the American Association of Anesthetists in Chicago after his return from the front in 1918 is typical[11]. He spoke of the volunteers in the McGill no.3 General Military Hospital who included specialists in surgery, medicine, ophthalmology, otorhinolaryngology, neurology, including an anæsthetist, as well as medical students.

Other war-time accounts describe how donations enabled an Ohio monovalve gas and oxygen apparatus to be purchased for the front in France. Details of the wounded; the fractures, contusions, shock and hæmorrhage are interspersed with descriptions of the delights of the beautiful countryside. Recipes are given for suitable general and local anæsthetics under battle conditions and on long marches using open drop ethyl chloride, ether and chloroform or cocaine, stovaine, novocaine and sedation with morphine and quinine-urea hydrochloride. Blood transfusion, seldom considered before, was extraordinarily successful in saving lives which otherwise would have been lost through exsanguination. Harvey Cushing gained unique experience in the treatment of penetrating head injury. He recognized that stabilization of the blood pressure of these trauma victims was crucial to survival if general anæsthesia was to be employed. Arthur E. Guedel (1883-1956), an anæsthetist

---

[10] Dr. William Boyman Howell was the grandson of Archdeacon Leach, a former McGill professor of classics and Vice-Principal of the University. Before the war, Dr. Howell was on the teaching staff of the Physiology Department and in private anæsthetic practice. He served as a major in the Canadian Army Medical Corps and became the chief anæsthetist at the Royal Victoria Hospital in Montreal after returning to Canada in 1918. He held this position until his retirement in 1937, when he and his wife moved to England.

[11] Howell, W.B. "Experiences of an anæsthetist at the front." *Quarterly Supplement of Anesthesia and Analgesia. American Journal of Surgery* 1918;116-7.

from Indianapolis, was among those who contrived ingenious devices, using foot bellows and rubber tubing, for the delivery of ether and air in a controlled manner, under the most difficult of conditions.

The invaluable knowledge contrived quickly and spontaneously on the battlefield would benefit many patients when the war ended. Research was now needed to further the techniques and treatments that were born of necessity. These objectives could not be met without considerable organization of the specialty. Appreciation for the McGill war effort brought the means to realize this research goal in the form of the Carnegie Foundation's $1 million gift to the Royal Institution in 1918 and the same amount from the Rockefeller Foundation to the faculty of medicine in 1920.

In 1918, Dr. Nagle died tragically from carbon monoxide poisoning[12]. The full-time hospital position was then offered to Wesley Bourne, but he refused this salaried appointment, preferring to continue his established private anæsthetic practice, which included St. Mary's Hospital, Western Hospital and Montreal Maternity Hospital, and later, the Royal Edward Hospital, Grace Dart Home and private dental practice.

---

[12] Dr. Nagle's death resulted from one of the first known cases of fatal inhalation of car exhaust fumes.

III

BETWEEN THE WARS (1918-39)

Montreal changed during the war. The Montreal Bicycling Club (the "Winged Wheelers") which had consisted mostly of officers in the militia, used to be a familiar sight riding in their uniforms around Côte-des-Neiges, Côte St. Luc and Mount Royal: it was disbanded when its members were called to serve in the war. However, their crest survived as the "Winged Wheel" of the Montreal Amateur Athletic Association and was later modified as the familiar crest of the Red Wings hockey team. Business lords, Lord Strathcona, Sir William Van Horne, Sir William MacDonald and others died. Most families lost at least one son. The financial empires were crumbling in the face of the introduction of income tax, and a lack of low-paying domestic help during the Depression years forced many families to abandon their Square Mile mansions.[1] McGill eventually acquired twelve of these to serve as classrooms and offices to cope with increasing enrolment: Allan's house "Ravenscrag" (hospital wing), Baumgarten's (Faculty Club), Davis' (Purvis Hall), Hosmer's (Physical and Occupational Therapy), Ross' (Chancellor Day Hall), Angus' (Conservatory of Music), Meredith's (Medicine, Ethics and Law), Wood's "Braehead" and Focher's (incorporated into the university), J.K.L. Ross' house site property (McIntyre Medical Sciences Building), Tiffin's house site property (Royal Victoria College), Joseph's "Dilcoosha" site property (McLennan Library).

McGill was a private university and benefitted from these events[2]. Colonel Herbert Molson gave the Molson Stadium to the University in memory of his brother, and J.W. McConnell, owner of the Montreal Star, donated $15

---

[1] MacKay, D. *The Square Mile. Merchant Princes of Montreal.* Vancouver, Toronto: Douglas and McIntyre Ltd., 1987.

[2] McGill traditionally received donations from well-known benefactors. Perhaps the most generous of these was the eccentric tobacco magnate Sir William Christopher Macdonald, who donated almost $15 million to McGill during his lifetime. His donations included student bursaries and funds to build a new chemistry building in 1887. In 1889 he gave a bequest towards the Macdonald Engineering Building, followed in 1891 with an endowed chair in electrical engineering and a large sum to the Faculty of Law. Macdonald College at Ste Anne de Bellevue, on the West Island was one of his largest gifts and was incorporated in 1906. He remained closely tied to the University, becoming Chancellor in 1914. Wesley Bourne regarded Macdonald as the greatest of the University's benefactors and used to tell his sons that he would probably have given even more to the University if the administration had been prepared to change its name from McGill to his own. His name is perpetuated in the rural college which he established only a year before Wesley Bourne entered the Faculty of Medicine.

million during his time as governor. The university was on the verge of a new era. Montreal's population had more than doubled (to 700,000) in the decade since Wesley Bourne's arrival and the community was changing: British numbers remained at a fairly constant level, but the French were now in the majority and multi-racial immigration was increasing. Jewish immigration was conspicuous for the first time and McGill limited the number of Jewish students by imposing higher academic entry requirements and a quota system. With the end of the war, despite the losses of life, the enrolment at McGill was fifty percent higher than before. This was due, to a large extent, to McGill's Khaki Army efforts which ensured that those in the armed forces had the opportunity to continue their education. Some may well have had less education in civilian life. With the return of war veterans, students numbered 3,000 in 1920. In fact, Canada was becoming an independent country, rather than a British colony. It became obvious that the medical faculty had to reorganize to accommodate a growing student population and changing needs.

Osler had maintained his connections with his alma mater and wrote persuasively to the Dean, General Herbert S. Birkett, urging him that:

> McGill cannot afford to fall behind other first-class medical schools...New conditions have arisen, to meet which it is essential to have sympathetic and active co-operation of the university and hospitals...which will involve a change of heart as to methods etc. and a realization of the full responsibility of the hospitals in this matter.

His advice, a reflection of his career goals, was based on the philosophy that viewed teaching, research and clinical care as closely linked. The difference was that he was now able to convince the administration that medical research must be integrated into all future plans for development of the medical faculty. Sir William Osler was a bibliophile, with a lifetime collection of 8,000 books in his library at the time of his death in 1919. He bequeathed most of his library to McGill, but it had to be catalogued before leaving Oxford, England, where Osler had been Regius Professor. This task was formidable and it took several years to produce the *Bibliotheca Osleriana*, before the collection was opened in 1929 in the Strathcona Medical Building. Here, it became the foundation of the flourishing Osler Library History of Medicine collection, now in the McIntyre Medical Sciences Building. The Osler Library for medical students had its beginnings in 1921. As a recent graduate, moving into his most productive years, Wesley Bourne shared Osler's attitudes.

Some outward signs of change were apparent. The right to bear a coat of arms was granted to McGill by King George V on 14th January, 1922, in response to the request of Sir Donald Alexander Smith, Baron Strathcona and Mount Royal. Prior to this, the University made use of the coat of arms of James McGill (1744-1813) its founder, which consisted of three white martlets, heraldic birds without beaks or feet, on a red background surmounted by a crown. Two mottoes were written across: *In domino confido,* after James McGill, and *Grandescunt aucta labore,* an old college motto. The personal arms were replaced by the present design, which more closely conforms to heraldic tradition. The red and white of James McGill's arms are reversed and the imperial crown has been removed. The red line dividing the shield represents the three peaks of Montreal's mountain, the book depicts learning, the two crowns, achievement. Use of the coat of arms is now protected by law, but some examples of the early "crest" are evident on Wesley Bourne's correspondence with the University. The appearance of the campus changed in 1925 with the erection of the distinctive Roddick Gates, of a classical Greek portico design, to replace an old wooden structure at the Sherbrooke Street entrance. They were erected in memory of Sir Thomas Roddick by his widow, to commemorate his contributions to McGill and Canadian medicine.

Within the Faculty of Medicine, the health sciences were foremost in importance and instruction was based on clinical training in the four teaching hospitals: the Montreal General Hospital, the Royal Victoria Hospital, the Montreal Children's Hospital and the Montreal Neurological Institute. The importance of the basic medical sciences, anatomy, pathology and pharmacology in the same faculty appeared to be complimentary, but conflicted with the relevance of related subjects, such as botany and zoology which were included in the science faculty. Research had to cross these artificial faculty boundaries. Appointments of faculty in more than one department were not unusual. Faculty organization was addressed promptly, with academic appointments accorded full or part-time status and designated by rank ranging from assistant to full professorships, tenable for one to three year terms. Tenure was not yet available, but pension reform resulted in a contributory scheme which was in place by 1929. This was offset by salary cuts for academics during the economic depression in 1932. Working relationships were formalized between the teaching hospitals and the university.

These trends were reflected in Wesley Bourne's faculty appointments recorded in his McGill staff record. Although he continued his private anæsthetic practice, his academic interests were intense and he was one of the first to apply basic sciences to the study of anæsthesia, working with Professor H.G. Barbour and Dr. R.L. Stehle in the Department of Pharmacology. In 1921 he was appointed Lecturer in Pharmacology at $100 per annum. This salary soon doubled, but in 1926 was abruptly reduced to $50. At some point he was re-categorized as Lecturer in Anæsthesia: noted as 1927 in his salary record and 1936 in his letter of appointment. In any event, his own loyalties were equally divided between these departments and he listed "Lecturer, Pharmacology-Anæsthesia McGill, 1921 - date" as his teaching appointments, when he completed the questionnaire for the 1940 *Directory of the American Society of Anesthetists Inc.* After ten years of service, he fared no better financially, being paid only $22.50 in 1933; with no remuneration thereafter. He was fortunate to receive even this derisory amount, as explained in a letter from the University administration[3]:

January Fifth 1934

Dr. Wesley Bourne
2310 Dorechester Street West,
Montreal

Dear Dr. Bourne,

Last Summer when reductions were being made in the budget of the Department of Pharmacology it was decided to discontinue the honorarium of $45, which was paid to you annually. I was not at that meeting and in that way you were not notified of this.

Under the circumstances I think the University should pay you for

---

[3] Wesley's son, Douglas, who now lives in Ottawa, did not recognize this address at 2310 Dorchester Street West, Montreal. He said that the family was living on Holton Avenue in Westmount at that time, but he knew that Dr. C.R. Bourne had an address on Dorchester Street. He thinks that this is most likely to be the original address of St. Mary's hospital, one of the hospitals where Wesley Bourne administered anæsthetics in his private practice, which started out in the mansion on Dorchester Street belonging to the Canadian Pacific Railway President, Lord Shaughnessy.

the first term, that is $22.50.

Please let me know if this is satisfactory to you.

Yours faithfully,

Secretary ...

His eldest son, Douglas, reported that his father, like many medical practitioners, was a bit naive about money. Wesley Bourne believed that if one did one's work well, there was no need to worry and that the money would take care of itself. Even though the family was going through financially difficult times, this did not deter Wesley Bourne from pursuing his goals. He continued to attend meetings, even though it was customary for guest lecturers to pay their own travel costs. John and Douglas attended Selwyn House School, a private boys' school, during the early years of the Depression. This meant that their father had to borrow money from his insurance to make it possible. Education for the children was his first priority and he probably jeopardized his own retirement plan to finance their education. He left most money matters to his wife, who managed their affairs very well under the circumstances. Fortunately, she had a good business head and was capable of dealing with the bank manager when he wanted to restrict the overdraft. Later on, when John was old enough to look after his father's books, he would send out bills to patients and follow up any deliquent payers. None of this really worried Wesley Bourne as he was not the slightest bit interested in money: his work was all that mattered.

The first Directory of Anesthetists, published in the *Anesthesia Supplement* in April, 1920, showed Dr. F.H. McMechan as secretary-treasurer of the American Association of Anesthetists, and listed Wesley Bourne of 42, St. Mark's Street, Montreal[4], in its membership. There were one hundred and seventy four anæsthetists, of which eight were from Canada (W. Bourne, G.M. Geldert, T.R. Hanley, W.G. Hepburn, W.B. Howell, S. Johnston, C. LaRocque and F.M. Nagle, then deceased). The number of anæsthetists in North America,

[4] This reference to 42 St. Mark's Street (*Quarterly Supplement of Anesthesia and Analgesia. American Journal of Surgery*, 1920;34:61-3) must have been a printer's error as the family lived at number 34 St. Mark's Street. The latter was the same address given for Wesley Bourne, as secretary of the Canadian Society of Anæsthetists, in the 1923 issue of the same journal (*Quarterly Supplement of Anesthesia and Analgesia. American Journal of Surgery*, 1923;37:29).

was now sufficient to warrant organization into societies. McMechan become the driving force behind several national societies which were established in the 1920s as umbrella organizations for regional societies set up to promote annual congresses where all interested North American anæsthetists could congregate and exchange ideas. The growth of these societies encouraged contacts between North American and British anæsthetists and was the impetus needed to promote the professionalism of anæsthesia.

The National Anesthesia Research Society began in 1919 with a mandate to promote science, education and the practice of anæsthesia. At its first meeting in Columbus, Ohio, in October 1922, Wesley Bourne gave an address on "Teaching of anæsthesia at McGill." Three years later (1925), this society had evolved into the more research-oriented International Anesthesia Research Society. The first issue of their publication *Current Researches in Anesthesia and Analgesia*, in 1922, included an article entitled "Morbidity and mortality in obstetrics as influenced by anesthesia" by Wesley Bourne. The Associated Anesthetists of the United States, formed in 1924 from the twelve-year-old American Association of Anesthetists, was later replaced by the American Society of Anesthesiologists and Canadian Anæsthetists' Society. After Wesley Bourne gave his presidential address to the fourth annual meeting of the combined Congress of Anesthesiologists of the United States, the Canadian Society of Anæsthetists and International Anesthesia Research Society, in Atlantic City in 1925, the Canadian society presented him with a silver loving cup and scroll of recognition for his research contributions.

Stimulated by McMechan's efforts, the original Canadian Society of Anæsthetists was started in 1920, with Wesley Bourne, at thirty-four years of age, as its secretary and treasurer. Bourne chose the emblem of the Canadian Society of Anæsthetists and its motto, attributable to Dean Moyse, "We watch closely those who sleep," written in the Greek form *Καθεύδοντας παρατηροὺμεν* (katheudontas parateroumen). This is emblazoned across the seal, which depicts the god Hypnos in the Cave of Sleep. By his feet are poppies, used to produce sleep, and Scottish thistles for awakening. This symbolism may have related more to practical matters than to affectionate acknowledgement of the artist's native country's close ties to the beginnings of anæsthesia. It seems that Wesley Bourne had commissioned A. Sheriff Scott (who later painted portraits of Wesley Bourne and Harold Griffith), a struggling young artist from Scotland, to design the emblem for the society. Bourne asked Scott to put the poppies on one side and bits of bark on the other. When it was finished, the artist told him that he had included a thistle and hoped that he would not mind, considering his Scottish origin. He went on to point out that anæsthetists might find it quite appropriate, as a thistle could be useful when waking the patient! Later, in writing his book *Mysterious Waters to Guard*, Wesley Bourne could not resist moralizing on the pertinence to anæsthesia of the mythological Cave of Sleep. This cave never admitted sunlight and reminded him of Ovid's tale of the drowsy House of Sleep.

> Near the land of the Cimerians there is a deep recess
> within a hollow mountain, the home and chamber of sluggish Sleep.
> Phoebus can never enter there with his rising, noontide, or setting rays,
> Clouds of vapour breathe forth from the earth, and dusky
> twilight shadows. There no wakeful, crested cock
> with his loud crowing summons dawn; no careful
> watch-dog breaks the silence with his voice, or goose,
> still shrewder than the dog. There is no sound
> of wild beast or of cattle, of branches rustling
> in the breeze, no clamorous tongues of men. There
> mute silence dwells. But from the bottom
> of the cave there flows the stream of Lethe, whose waves,
> gently murmuring over the gravelly bed, invite to slumber.
> Before the cavern's entrance abundant poppies bloom,
> and countless herbs, from whose juices dewy night
> distils sleep and spreads its influence over the darkened lands.
>
> (After Ovid, *Metamorphosis* XI 592-607)

The inaugural meeting of the Canadian Society of Anæsthetists in Niagara Falls, Ontario, was held jointly with the Interstate Association of Anesthetists, the New York Society of Anesthetists and the Ontario Medical Association in June, 1921. This forum provided an opportunity to debate the current issues in anæsthesia, as shown by the programme contents. Clinical matters predominated, with Wesley Bourne contributing his talk on the effect of anæsthesia on morbidity and mortality in obstetrics. Other topics included anæsthesia for brain surgery, tonsillectomies and the effects of ether, nitrous oxide, and ethyl chloride on the circulation and liver. Guedel presented his observations on the classification of anæsthetic signs of ethyl chloride anæsthesia in man, which was soon to be followed by publication of his classical descriptions of the stages in anæsthesia[5]. Important political views of anæsthestic practice were addressed in talks titled "Anæsthesia—its place in the practice of medicine" and "The medical profession and the nurse anæsthetist."

The Society did not last. In 1928 it was disbanded in favour of an Anæsthetic Section in affiliation with the Canadian Medical Association. There were systemic problems, inherent in maintaining an independent society with only one hundred members and a handful of full-time practitioners, may have been important, some blamed Wesley Bourne for the failure because "The society elected a secretary who did not write letters."[6]. Nevertheless, the members continued to be active and the Montreal Society of Anæsthetists was formed in 1930, largely due to the persistence of Harold R. Griffith, by this time a close friend and colleague of Wesley Bourne.

Bourne and Griffith were also members of an elite group known as the Anesthetists' Travel Club. Their inaugural meeting was held in 1930 in Madison, Wisconscin, where Ralph Waters had established the first academic department with a residency training programme. The following year the Travel Club had twenty-two members eight of whom were Canadian. A final meeting took place in 1942 in Montreal and then the annual gatherings lapsed. However, Harold Griffith saw this group as critical to the international dissemination of information on the state of anæsthesia. With renewed vigour, the Travel Club members re-grouped in 1952 to set up plans for the establishment of the World Federation of Societies of Anæsthesiologists. Thus, the common bonds among Canada's anæsthetists continued to grow, until they were ready to leave the Montreal-based society behind and move on to the formation of the new Canadian Anæsthetists' Society in 1943.

Bourne was active as a member of the Society of Sigma X (1922), the Montreal Medico-Chirurgical Society, the Montreal Physiological Society, the Canadian Physiological Society (1935), the Canadian Medical Association, American Society for Experimental Therapeutics (1936) and as a corresponding member of the Royal Society of Medicine (1926), Société Française

---

[5] Guedel, A.E. "Third stage ether anesthesia: a sub-classification regarding the significance of the position and movements of the eyeball." *Quarterly Supplement of Anesthesia and Analgesia. American Journal of Surgery*, 1920;34:53-5.

[6] Gordon, R.A. "A capsule history of anæsthesia in Canada." *Canadian Anæsthetists Society Journal*, 1978;25:75-83.

d'Anesthésie et d'Analgésie (1935), the Association of Anæsthetists of Great Britain and Ireland, the Associated Anesthetists of the United States and Canada, and the British Medical Association. He was pivotal to the development of many of these societies and held office in their organizations:

1922	Research Committee, National Anesthesia Research Society
1924-5	President, Associated Anesthetists of United States and Canada
1920-4	Secretary-Treasurer, Canadian Society of Anæsthetists
1925	President, International Aneasthesia Reserach Society
1932-6	President, Section on Anæsthesia, Canadian Medical Association
1932	Vice-president and Secretary, Anæsthesia Section, British Medical Association Centeneray Meeting, London, England
1940	President, International Anesthesia Research Society
1942	President, American Society of Anesthesiologists

Formalisation and standardization of education were gradually having an effect on the medical curriculum. At McGill the medical course was modified in September, 1936 to provide for a minimum of five years professional training leading to the MD CM degree, and one year of approved internship or additional study in a medical school setting[7]. This consolidated training into a five-year period, one year less than it had been in the previous program.

The Royal College of Physicians and Surgeons of Canada was established in 1929 with Wesley Bourne, who held a fellowship in internal medicine from 1931, as one of its charter fellows. The College was a regulatory body which granted specialty fellowship diplomas by examination. It mattered little whether this diploma was a prerequisite for being a specialist, which many physicians already considered themselves to be, or an academic trademark; fellowship status was denied to anæsthetists. Recognition as a specialty was important as negotiations for fees and hospital positions came to depend on such credentials. The Diploma in Anæsthetics (DA) marked official recognition of the specialty in Great Britain in 1935 and the United States followed in 1938. Consequently, Canadian anæsthetists were frustrated in their attempts to seek professional status just prior to the Second World War.

[7] "University notes. McGill University: reorganization of the medical course." *Canadian Medical Association Journal*, 1936;34:340-41.

Wesley Bourne's career began vigorously and he achieved many major accomplishments during the two decades between the wars. He possessed an enormous capacity for both work and play. How he found time, beyond his teaching, research, organizational and administrative activities (to say nothing of his regular private anæsthetic practice) for so much recreation, remains a mystery to his family. All of these activities were undertaken obsessively, with contagious enthusiasm. He was an avid clubman. His main social club was the University Club, in addition to the Faculty Club, where he spent many evenings socializing with friends like Stephen Leacock. He was also an enthusiastic member of the Winchester Fishing Club, the Kanawaki Golf Club and a curling club on Boulevard de Maisonneuve (formerly St Luke's Street, between Guy Street and Atwater Avenue). He was a considerable sportsman, golfer, angler, gardener and, in later years, photographer. The small garden at his home at 32, Holton Avenue had two of the most resplendent flower beds on the street. Wesley Bourne grew two varieties of morning glory (heavenly blue and Scarlett O'Hara) and each morning he would send his son out to count the number of blooms and report the total. One day he asked John to remove the dead heads from the petunias and was furious on finding that he had removed a lot of unopened buds. From then on John was only allowed to help with the Spring and Fall digging.

He read a great deal and was seldom seen without a book in his hand. His sons would collect the books he had reserved in the Redpath Library in Redpath Hall. He read everything from light novels to the profoundest of philosophers; being particularly fond of the works of John Ruskin and Thomas Babbington Macaulay's Histories. As he read, he always made notes. Not infrequently, his son Robert would arrive home late at night and find him asleep with his glasses askew on his head and a book on his chest. One night, as he was turning out the light, he saw that the book was written in Greek on one page and there was a translation into English on the opposite page. Wesley Bourne would often use obscure quotations when talking or writing, prompting one of his good friends and co-researcher, Nicholas Dyer, to give him the name "Viselius"; Dyer in turn being called "Aristophanes," the comic poet. This characteristic humour was reminiscent of Osler, who wrote pseudonymously as Egerton Y. Davis. Wesley Bourne had a great interest in languages and at various times undertook the study of French, German, Spanish and Russian. Initially, he devoted considerable time to learning languages, but was never able to master them fully because of the general pressure of other occupations.

His introduction to fishing was the result of an invitation from a Dr. and Mrs. Argue to stay in pension at McGregor Lake, located between Montebello and Ottawa, north of the Ottawa River. Mr. Douglas Haines, also an invited guest, was an employee of the Canadian Pacific Railway. His duties included entertaining visitors by taking them fishing at the fishing and hunting lodges owned by the company. This first morning before breakfast, Haines asked the party to join him to see if they could catch some bass for breakfast. On his first cast from the dock, with bait, casting rod and lure, he caught a three-pound black bass which put up a great fight. Wesley Bourne could not wait to get back to Montreal and immediately equipped himself with rods and tackle. This was when he joined his fishing and hunting club, the Winchester Club. After that, the family would go there once a year for a week or so in July and had a wonderful time. This was relaxing for Bourne as he loved the Canadian woods and the French-Canadian folk songs sung by the guides.

One of his sons, Robert, visited his father frequently at McGill's Department of Pharmacology. Once, he noticed a small cot made up as a bed beside the laboratory bench. His father told him that this was where he slept when he needed to test blood samples throughout the night for his experiments. In later life, Robert asked him how he could work all day administering anæsthetics, be on call for twenty-four hours, yet still find time for his all-consuming research. Wesley Bourne's reply explained much about him: "Research was always my fun. I always looked forward to it, just as you look forward to sports after you have finished your work." In retrospect, his "Fun", his "Research," was the singular trait that distinguished him from most of the other pioneer anæsthetists of that time.

In the 1930s, Wesley Bourne was one of the few (Beecher and Rovenstine were others) who saw beyond the technical limits of anæsthesia. However, communication of information about new anesthetic drugs and techniques, clinical observations, research findings, teaching, service organization and departmental administration depended on routine attendance at meetings and conference proceedings. The Montreal *Gazette* published reports of his lectures to local group meetings. On 3rd May, 1933 and 8th January, 1934 he gave talks to the Rotary Club in the Windsor Hotel and the Young Men's Association of the St. Laurent United Church. Both talks delivered the same message, that anæsthesia had been made safe and should not be feared. In fact, the press gave Bourne's department considerable attention; the *Montreal Star* showing photographs of him lecturing to a group of visiting doctors from

Wisconsin. As most of the presentations were fully written and read verbatim, it was easy to report the proceedings of these meetings to a wider audience through publication in journals and newsletters. Wesley Bourne first published in the Canadian Medical Association journal and some of the regional medical journals, until anæsthetic societies flourished and the number of their own journals increased. His contributions could be found in the following journals, which appeared during his career:

1922	*Current Researches in Anesthesia and Analgesia* in 1957 became: *Anesthesia and Analgesia, Current Researches* in 1979 became: *Anesthesia and Analgesia*
1923	*British Journal of Anesthesia*
1935	*Anésthesie et Analgésie*
1939	*Revista Argentina de Anestesiologia*
1940	*Anesthesiology*
1946	*Anæsthesia*
1952	*Der Anæsthetist*
1954	*Canadian Anæsthetists' Society Journal* In 1987 became: *Canadian Journal of Anæsthesia/Journal Canadien d'Anesthésie*

The late appearance of *Anesthesiology* in 1940, the journal of the largest specialist body, the American Society of Anesthesiologists (preceded by the American Society of Anesthetists Inc. which existed from 1936-1944) is perplexing until it is realized that Paul Wood, secretary-treasurer of the society, had an agreement with F. McMechan that prevented its earlier publication. This agreement did not allow other publications while *Current Researches in Anesthesia and Analgesia* was in existence. As the agreement was limited to the period of McMechan's editorship, the society was released from this undertaking upon his death in 1939 and was free to publish its own journal[8]. Speculation that the American Society of Anesthetists Inc/American Society of Anesthesiologists and the International Anesthesia Research Society would amalgamate, or produce a combined journal, was not realized. However, both

[8] Bacon, D.R. "The promise of one great society. The 1939-40 proposed merger of the American Society of Anesthetists and the International Anesthesia Research Society." *Anesthesiology*, 1994;80:929-35.

organizations have flourished independently, free of the controlling influence of McMechan, although indebted to him for their inception.

In the period between the wars Wesley Bourne was at his most productive. From 1926-30 he travelled widely, giving invited lectureships. He attended meetings and congresses in Montreal, Winnipeg, Columbus (Ohio), Chicago, Ottawa, Atlantic City, Glasgow, Toronto, Washington DC, Boston, Philadelphia, London (England), New York, Calgary, Rochester, Halifax and Hot Springs, Vermont. He appealed to a surprisingly wide audience, and was invited to speak to groups of nurses, hospital administrators, medical students, obstetricians, pharmacologists and physiologists, as well as anæsthetists across North America. Given the need to reach as large an audience as possible, the same paper would often be published simultaneously in two journals. These presentations evolved into over one hundred articles in twelve journals published at the time.

The themes of research, clinical anæsthesia, teaching and administration flow through all of his productive period, although the emphasis changed as his career advanced. In this first twenty years, he published almost entirely on research and clinical anæsthesia, reflecting his own interests and involvements during the time. Anæsthesia found new challenges in lung surgery, the treatment of thyroid goitre, Pott's disease of the spine, surgery in diabetics and its application at the extremes of age; heralding the popular use of tracheal intubation and artificial ventilation. The teaching of anæsthesia to medical students was effected quite early, but there was a shift in the late 1930s towards hospital administration and the organization of anæsthesia services. His research into physiological derangements during anæsthesia concentrated on temperature regulation, shifts of body fluids and electrolytes, metabolic effects of ether, acetaldehyde, morphine, sodium amytal and the effects of anæsthesia on the liver and kidneys. All of these were supported by careful clinical observations in large numbers of patients. Wesley Bourne recognized the problems confronting clinicians and sought their causes and remedies as he investigated the bodily effects of anæsthetic agents which were only just being appreciated by the scientific community.

These manuscripts are now part of the archives of medicine and can be read in their entirety. However, much of the clinical practice therein is now of historical interest since the pharmaceutical industry has produced a new storehouse of more potent and expensive drugs for the anæsthetist to explore.

The research methodology, too, has been superseded as chemical and mechanical methods of investigation have given way to modern biotechnological advances, microcellular probing and computerization of data collection. Nevertheless, these articles provide insight into the foundations of modern anesthesia in Canada, in particular its development at McGill. More intriguing, would be to read them for Wesley Bourne's sense of "Fun" and appreciate his easy use of words derived from Greek and Latin, his effortless interjection of philosophical works, mastery of English literature, and perhaps criticize his occasional lapse into pomposity. To digress: a selection of a few apt quotations from the publications of his most active period are chosen to illustrate Wesley Bourne's comprehension of all facets of anæsthesia, research[9], clinical anæsthesia[10], teaching[11] and administration[12] and the interdependence of these individual aspects of the specialty.

In reporting his research, Bourne provided a model which has not been bettered since. Instead of an abstract to lay the roadmap through the study, he fashioned a summarizing concluding paragraph which served the same purpose. All of his work was original, building on current and contemporary concepts introduced by a small number of scientists. He described the problem and the means to its solution succinctly, and proposed conclusions drawn clearly from his findings. Summaries of these study results were often the main theme of his addresses to congresses. His teaching was always based on his extensive clinical

---

[9] On research: "The purpose of the experiments to be described was to obtain further light upon the interrelations between the alkali reserve and hydrogen ion concentration of the blood and the sodium and potassium content of the urine during anesthesia produced by ether alone, as well as by ether and morphine together." (*J Biol Chem* 1922;53:341-8).

[10] On clinical anæsthesia: "In the technique of administering nitrous oxide ... a thorough knowledge of the apparatus to be used, and there are many satisfactory ones available; an ample suppy of nitrous oxide and oxygen; careful methods of induction of anæsthesia, such as the avoidance of sensations of suffocation; a complete acquaintance with the signs of anæsthesia, which signs are very definite with nitrous oxide." (*Canadian Medical Association Journal*, 1923;13:50).

[11] On teaching: "To advance anæsthesia in medicine we believe that those interested in the subject must do more research work and better teaching. The quality of the latter is affected by the former." (*British Journal of Anæsthesia*, 1923;1:74-8 and *Current Researches in Anesthesia and Analgesia*, 1923;2:197-9).

[12] On administration: "To us it is particularly encouraging to note the increasing interest shown by the majority of students, some of whom are now asking to be admitted as house anæsthetists at graduation. This should offer a real solution to the difficulty in obtaining qualified graduates in medicine to administer anæsthetics." (*British Journal of Anæsthesia* 1923;1:74-8).

experience as a practising anæsthetist, together with his well known understanding approach and strong empathy with patients. More importantly, he sought to examine these clinical practices carefully. Although teaching medical students was an adjunct to his clinical practice, he was quick to point out to them the necessity for constant enquiry and clinical observation. He was perceptive enough to realize that it would not be possible to be as involved in the future of anæsthesia as he wanted, without devoting considerable time and thought to the organization of the specialty and its societies, and to the delivery of anæsthetic services in an institutional setting as well as in private practice.

Dr. E.J. Chambers of Doncaster, England, was one of those who visited Wesley Bourne at the Royal Victoria Hospital in Montreal to watch him adminstering anæsthesia[13]. He wanted to know the best way to produce abdominal relaxation using the nitrous oxide and oxygen technique and was able to see a variety of approaches, using the Gwathmey-Foregger and McKesson machines. Bourne always gave sound clinical advice and warned against allowing cyanosis to occur, while adding carbon dioxide and some ether to the nitrous oxide mixture. All was explained in simple terms, just as he would have done for a large audience at meetings of the societies.

The vexing question of who would be responsible for administering anæsthesia was never as great an issue in Canada as south of the border. However, there were increasing demands for service which made the physician-anæsthetist quite vulnerable. Bourne's attitude towards this was to educate nurses in anæsthesia so that they were well informed, but he stopped short of encouraging them to have a role in the administration of anæsthesia. He made his views clear at an American College of Surgeons meeting:

> Concerning legal responsibility, there is little to be said. The law as to who may administer anesthetics varies in different countries and in various states. In Canada, no one may give anesthetics but a qualified practitioner of medicine and surgery. As to whether the surgeon or the anesthetist is responsible, it would seem to be simply this: that if the anesthetist is a qualified physician he is just as responsible for the administration of anesthetic drugs as he is for administering any other

---

[13] Chambers, E.J. "The story of a journey in search of information." *British Journal of Anæsthesia*, 1927-8;5:158-66.

drugs. The surgeon becomes responsible if he employs any one who does not hold a license to practice medicine in the locality in which the anesthetic is given." (*Hospital Management* 1938;46:39-41).

This controversy was settled in 1938, at least in Canada, as a result of a case at one of Wesley Bourne's own hospitals, the Royal Victoria in Montreal[14]. The widow of a patient, Mr. F.J. McFall, who died on the operating table, claimed damages against Dr. Turner, the surgeon who employed Nurse Butler to administer a gas and oxygen anæsthetic. The Supreme Court held that the death could not be attributed to the nurse. On the other hand, the court found that the hospital and the surgeon were at fault for allowing a non-physician to administer the anæsthetic: "...the surgeon cannot, and should not supervise the anæsthesia, that is not his business, all his attention and his faculties should be concentrated on the operation itself...the anæsthetist is, therefore, the only person who watches the patient, actually and completely."

In his later publications, Bourne wrote as much to amuse himself as to enthrall his audience. A more philosophical approach emerged and titles such as "The perfecting of anæsthesia," "Anæsthesia for the Republic of Plato," and "Fors clavigera in anæsthesia" masked the mundane. Superficial reading allows some perplexity as to the meaning and relevance of the frequent allusions. It is only on reflection, and with greater understanding of his superb mastery of the English language and use of quotations from the classics, that the subtle and deliberate intent of these metaphors can be appreciated and the true inferences revealed.

Wesley Bourne received his Master of Science (MSc) degree in 1922 (the first anæsthetist ever to do so) for his thesis on heart regulation, water exchange and ether. Widespread recognition for his achievements followed. He was elected to the presidency of the International Anesthesia Research Society in 1925 and passed the gavel to his successor, Dr. John H. Evans in 1926. At the annual dinner during the third annual Congress of Anesthetists in Los Angeles in 1925 he received one of his greatest accolades from Dr. F.H. McMechan[15]. In appreciation for his research and contributions to the organization of the speciality, the secretary-general presented him with a silver

---

[14] "Casual Comments." *British Journal of Anæsthesia*, 1938;16:142-4.

[15] "A builder of bridges." *Current Researches in Anesthesia and Analgesia*, 1925;4:130.

loving cup and alluded to him as "a builder of bridges," quoting this poem, "The Bridge Builder" by Will Allen Dromgoole[16].

> A traveller, going a lone highway,
> Came at the evening, cold and gray,
> To a chasm vast and deep and wide,
> The traveller crossed in the twilight dim,
> The sullen stream had no fear from him;
> But he turned when safe on the other side
> And built a bridge to span the tide.
> 'My friend,' said a fellow pilgrim near,
> 'You are wasting your strength with building here:
> Your journey will end with the ending day,
> You never again will pass this way;
> You've crossed the chasm deep and wide:
> Why build you this bridge at eventide?'
> 'Good friend, in the path I have come,' he said
> 'There followeth after me today,
> A youth whose feet must pass this way,
> This chasm that has been as nought to me
> To that fair-haired youth may a pitfall be:
> He too must cross in the twilight dim -
> Good friend, I am building this bridge from him!'

Wesley Bourne was awarded the prize for the best essay in the *British*

---

[16] The title and authorship of the poem was not quoted in the original reference and almost proved to be elusive. Although not necessary for the completion of this biography of Wesley Bourne, it became a challenge to locate the poem in its original form. Searches in libraries from Montreal to Vancouver took many hours, even days, but yielded no information. Indices of first lines of poetry provided no clues and it seemed possible that it might be a portion from a larger work, making it less easy to identify. At least it had to be written before 1926, which limited the time frame of the search. Turning to computers, the internet listed some English poetry and frustrated entry into the definitive database form subscribers. Just as the might of the university departments of English at McGill and the University of British Columbia was to be applied to this task, the poem was found by Ms. Donna MacFarlane, the residency program secretary at the McGill Department of Anesthesia, in Montreal's Champlain College collection, but only after a very long search. The poem is "The Bridge Builder" by Will Allan Dromgoole (1865-1943) and it appeared in the book *The Best Loved Poems of the American People*, selected by Hazel Fellman and published by Doubleday and Company Inc, New York in 1936 as a tribute to Adolphe S. Ochs (1858-1935), the publisher of the *New York Times*.

Journal of Anæsthesia of 1934 for his paper, coauthored by B.B. Raginsky, on "Vinyl ether (vinesthene) anæsthesia in dogs: effects upon normal and impaired liver." This success was tainted somewhat by the judges comments: "They would have been happier, perhaps, if the winning essay had been of a nature to be of greater clinical or practical benefit....the exact nature of the subject matter was only one of the considerations to be taken into account in awarding merit, and those essays which in this particular were preferred to the winner were too far behind in other respects to displace it." (*Br J Anæsth* 1934-5;12:51). Given the experiences with chloroform hepatotoxicity (halothene hepatitis was not yet known), this is a fairly unenlightened viewpoint. Moreover, there were at least nine publications on experimentation with dogs in his laboratory which were directly related to the problem. Bourne had lamented as early as 1928, in addressing the Associate Anesthetists in Washington, DC, that anæsthetists were continuing to use chloroform on their patients even as its deleterious effects on the liver were becoming well recognized. However, he was awarded unreservedly, an honourable mention in the 1936 prize competition for his paper (with co-investigators S. Dworkin and B.B. Raginsky) on "Action des anesthésiques, sedatifs, hypnotiques sur les centres nerveux supérieurs" by the Société d'Anesthésia et d'Analgésie.

Recognition in England was also afforded in full to Wesley Bourne. In 1935, the Royal Society of Medicine made him the first recipient of the Hickman Medal, given for original and outstanding achievement in anæsthesia. Robert Bourne was ten years old, an impressionable age, at the time. He recalls the living room being full of reporters, photographers and flood lights for press interviews with his father for this special occasion. Dr. Hickman, an Edinburgh graduate, in 1822-4 showed that animals breathing carbon dioxide felt no pain. This convinced him of the value of "suspended animation" to produce insensibility during surgical operations on humans. Although he died more than a decade before nitrous oxide and ether were introduced, he is given credit for the "discovery" of anæsthesia. The award was made possible by the Henry Hill Hickman Memorial Committee's donation of £200 to establish a bronze medal to commemorate this physician's work. It is struck with a depiction of Hickman on one side and a representation of anæsthesia as a beautiful woman who has broken the chain tying a patient to the devil, pain, on the other. This medal is awarded at intervals of three years or more: going to Drs. Ivan W. Magill (London, England) in 1938, Arthur E. Guedel (Los Angeles, California) in 1941, Harold R. Griffith (Montreal, Canada) in 1956 and Philip Bromage (Montreal, Canada) in his retirement in 1987.

Wesley Bourne always seemed to know a little more about things than most: in his memorial address at the 1939 International College of Anesthetists joint meeting in Philadelphia, he pointed out the interesting connection between Francis H. McMechan and Henry Hill Hickman. Dr. McMechan's wife was formerly Laurette van Varseveld of Paris, France. She was a direct descendant of the sister of Baron Dominique Larrey, Napoleon's surgeon in chief who, in 1828, had supported Hickman's claims about suspended animation.

In 1938, Bourne was one of five Canadian anæsthetists to receive the English speciality Diploma in Anæsthetics (DA), without examination, under the enabling regulations. He also belonged to the International College of Anesthetists, which bestowed its fellowship diploma (FICA) on its members. This college was formed by Dr. Francis McMechan about 1938, close to his death in 1939, but it was never particularly relevant, and ceased after a decision taken at the World Federation of Society of Anæsthesiologists Interim Committee in 1953.

Despite his career distractions and an extraordinary dedication to the development of anæsthesia, Wesley Bourne enjoyed his young family and was keenly interested in his children's welfare and, in particular, their education. It was easy to see that he and his wife, Sara, were always close and, as with all great men, she was an enormous help to him through times of joy and trial. Some of his closest friends, who were household names in their home, were great anæsthetists or academics: Harold R. Griffith, M. Digby Leigh, Ralph Waters, Henry Barbour, Ivan W. Magill, Robert Macintosh and John Gillies. The world community of anæsthestists was very closely knit at that time and Wesley Bourne enjoyed entertaining at home, so the family met all of these doctors. They would rave about the meals prepared by the Bourne's Chinese cook, Tom Gum Yet. Often the meal would be followed by a "sing-song" around the piano, which would include Bourne's favourite songs "Let me call you sweetheart" and "Beulahland."

In the good years, before the 1929 stock market crash and ensuing Depression, Bourne bought his suits from a Savile Row tailor who sent a representative to Montreal each year. Among other things, John says that his father was a bit of a "dandy" and was always extremely well-dressed, with ties and handkerchiefs to match. His shoes were always well polished, a job which he gave to his son.

Wesley Bourne's sons have fond memories of their father during this period between the wars. Robert and he were very close. They would work together in the garden, which was sometimes enjoyable for both, and his father encouraged Robert to read, which which for him is a source of enjoyment. In 1938, the two had season tickets for the football matches, even though Wesley Bourne knew little about the game. It was the year that the intercolliagate football championship game was held at McGill and he was pleased to go and share his son's enthusiasm for sports. John thought that his father was rather severe and strict with his older brother, Douglas, because Wesley was overly ambitious for his first son. He wanted Douglas to achieve academically, which he did. However, John's overall recollection was of a kind and gentle man.

At five years of age, while on holiday on the Maine Coast, his father helped John to overcome his fear of water, carrying him into the breakers himself. He realized that John was not much of a student and did not push him as much, although he did say "If you don't read you will never know anything; in fact you will be an ignoramus." His son now admits that he wishes that he had listened to his father, as he realizes how much he has missed by not being a reader. He also remembers a well-earned spanking when they were living on St Mark Street, close to the western division of the Montreal General Hosptial, now the Montreal Children's Hospital. The painters had just finished painting the garage doors in an off-white colour and there was a pan of refuse oil in the garage, so John decided to paint the doors again. When his father came home he was furious and sent John to his room without supper. Later that evening, he went to see John, obviously even more upset at these events that his son.

John and Douglas are both grateful for their father's encouragement to join the McGill University Canadian Officer's Training Corps (COTC) in the Fall of 1934. Douglas continued in the Royal Canadian Signals Corps, in line with his training as an electronics engineer. John remembers that when he was puzzling over which regiment to join, his father wisely recommended the Black Watch, the best choice John could have made. Wesley Bourne knew the Montreal regiments well as he commanded no. 9 Field Ambulance (RCAMC) which was part of the militia. Wesley enrolled them as junior members in his own club, the Kanawaki Golf Club. Golf not only gave them great pleasure, but introduced them to many friends that they would not have met otherwise.

Wesley treated Hilary Bourne, his nephew, like a son, and was always there for help and advice. He was responsible, along with his wife who was a

Montrealer, for Hilary living and practising medicine in Montreal. When Hilary qualified in medicine at McGill, Wesley Bourne said, "It is better for you to stay here and be a little fish in a big pond that to be a big fish in a little pond somewhere else." He was sincere about that, but added "The first thing you will have to do is to get rid of that 'gawd awful' Barbadian accent," the same remark made to him by the Dean of Medicine at McGill about thirty years earlier.

Paradoxically, these transitional years bewteen the wars were, perhaps, the best for Wesley Bourne. In the economic depression of the 1930s, when private practice was something of a luxury, he just spent more time having "fun" in his laboratory and his reputation grew steadily. During these pivotal two decades, he laid the foundations, not only for his own successes, but for the future of McGill Anesthesia.

Wesley Bourne's Association with Anæsthetic Societies

*still active in 1995

1893 London (Eng) Society of Anæsthetists
→1908-date Anæsthetic Section, Royal Society of Medicine*

1905 Long Island Society of Anestetists
→1911 New York Society of Anesthetists
→1936 American Society of Anesthetists Inc.
→1944 - date American Society of Anesthesiologists*

1912-24 American Association of Anesthetists = 1912 Scottish Society of Anesthetists, 1915 Interstate Association of Anesthetists, 1915 Mid-Western Asociation of Anesthetists (→Ohio State Medical Associaton→Pacific Coast Association→Anesthesia Section of California State Med Association), 1919 Brooklyn Society of Anesthetists
→1924-41 Associated Anesthetists of US & Canada = 1920 CSA, 1919 NARS, Eastern Society of Anesthetists, Mid-Western Association of Anesthetists, Pacific Coast Assoc of Anesthetists → replaced by ASA/CAS

1919-25 National Anesthesia Research Society
→ parent organization for Associated Anesthetists of US & Canada = 1922 New York Society of Anesthetists
→1925-date International Anæsthesia Research Society*

1920-28 Canadian Society of Anesthetists
→with Associated Anesthetists of US & Canada
→1928-30 Anesthesia Section, Canadian Medical Association
→1930-43 Montreal Society of Anesthetists
→1943-date Canadian Anæsthetists' Society*

1929-52 Anesthetists' Travel Club
→-date Academy of Anæsthesiologists*

IV

WARTIME CIRCUMSTANCES (1939-45)

Canada's declaration of war, on 10th September, 1939, one week after the British declaration, symbolized the spirit of independence developing in the country. Lessons had been learned from the 1914-18 war and blind allegiance within the Commonwealth was not forthcoming. Although conscription was rejected by Quebec in 1942, McGill expanded its Canadian officer training corps (COTC) from 125 to 1400 volunteers at the beginning of the war. The Faculty of Medicine organized two Canadian hospitals, numbers one and fourteen, which served in England, Sicily and Italy. In all, 5,500 graduates were registered with allied organizations. Nevertheless, McGill gave priority to maintaining the University's programmes in all departments as far as possible: a pivotal decision which facilitated the tremendous post-war developments.

In 1940, the principalship of McGill passed to thirty-six-year-old Frank Cyril James. He was the eleventh to hold the position, which he filled for the next twenty-two years. He came from a modest English background and had struggled to make his academic grades, but was successful in obtaining his PhD in economics at the University of Pennsylvania, before being invited to Montreal. His style of leadership was appropriate for this period: he was able to make decisions and could ignore unwanted advice. In these difficult times Quebec, a province led by the conservative Premier Duplessis and still dominated by the Roman Catholic Church, would foster the growth of McGill. Students delayed enlistment until they had completed their courses, ensuring that they could specialize during and after the war. Continuing teaching and research activities on campus turned to immediate and relevant needs: accelerated training for radio-technicians, nutritional research, food-growing techniques, biological assays for vitamins, special paper products, the manufacture of explosives, DDT and chemical warfare. The student body of 3,275 in 1939, increased somewhat to 3,905 by the Spring of 1945 and began to expand rapidly when the war ended. Returning veterans swelled the numbers to 6,370 by the Fall of 1945.

This was the era of "The Great Triumvirate" of McGill anæsthetists: Wesley Bourne, Harold Randall Griffith and Morton Digby Leigh. Wesley Bourne served as an honorary lieutenant colonel in the RCAMC, commanding the no. 9 Field Ambulance (which was part of the militia) for the duration of the war; the group acted as consultants to the Army, Navy and Air Force to teach anæsthesia for wartime use. The intensive four-month course in anæsthesia and the systematic training for officers which they developed for the armed forces, was based on the two-year graduate course started in the Montreal hospitals in 1940. This evolved into the formalized diploma course and residency training programme of the post-war McGill department. The first Canadian residency programme in anæsthesia had begun with three one-year internships in the Toronto hospitals in 1934, followed by one at the Royal Victoria Hospital in Montreal two years later. Dr. M. Digby Leigh attests to the humble beginnings of the prestigious McGill Annual Review Course and residency teaching programme in a letter, dated 7th February, 1966 to the librarian of the Wood Library Museum:

> Dear Mr. Necker,
>
> I left Madison, Wisconsin, after three excellent years with Dr. Ralph Waters and took a job at the Children's Memorial Hospital in Montreal in July, 1939. The salary finally agreed upon was $4,000.00 per annum. My first resident was sent by McGill University. Once a week this lone resident and I held a meeting to discuss our interesting cases. I invited other residents from the other hospitals to join us and some came.
>
> About 1943, when the Canadian Navy, Army and Air Force decided to send physicians for training in anesthesia, I fortunately had the opportunity of developing a three-month training course. Each resident rotated around the different hospitals for a couple of weeks. The group expanded, so (the) Ciba Company was persuaded to let us use its lecture hall in the building downtown. Interesting cases were presented from all over Montreal. Dr. Griffith then joined Dr. Bourne and me. Anæsthetists from all parts of Canada came for longer periods of training and a three year Diploma Course was formed. Since we were not recognized by McGill University, Dr. Bourne and I formed the Montreal College of Anæsthesia.........

The Ciba postgraduate course, as these meetings came to be known, was directed by Wesley Bourne and M. Digby Leigh and was a forum in which the French and English anæsthetists of the Montreal hospitals came together on a regular basis[1]. Georges Cousineau, Harold R. Griffith, R. Rochette, W. Tremblay and F.A.H. Wilkinson collaborated in producing the programme.

---

[1] Dr Georges Cousineau's original documents were found in a box of his papers by his nephew, Dr Jean-Pierre Tétrault, Directeur, Département d'anesthésie-réanimation, Université de Sherbrooke, Quebec.

Typewritten handouts were provided to cover twenty-six meetings which took place over twelve months, the last in February, 1944. Dr. Cousineau's original copy of the programme of the second meeting, dated 10th March, 1993 described five interesting cases and six deaths related to anæsthesia for discussion in the meeting. Anæsthesia included cyclopropane, the Etheringon-Wilson and Howard Jones spinal techniques with nupercaine or procaine. Complications were clearly described and possible causes openly discussed: laryngeal stricture following closure of a patent ductus arteriosus in a six-year-old girl; respiratory arrest during cyclopropane induction of anæsthesia after premedication with nembutal, morphine and atropine in a sixty-five-year-old patient scheduled for hysterectomy; hypotensive collapse after spinal anæsthesia, and seizures during cyclopropane anæsthesia in a fourteen-year-old boy[2]. Deaths occurred in elderly patients requiring emergency surgery, with diagnoses of acute appendicitis, perforated peptic ulcer, intestinal obstruction from volvulus and prostatatic obstruction. They were extremely ill before surgery was contemplated and were given spinal anæsthesia. Circulatory support was needed during the procedures, but all survived and died several hours or days later as a result of their medical and surgical problems: listed as hypotension, cardiac failure, toxæmia, intracranial hæmorrhage, pleural adhesions, kidney swelling, surgical bleeding and diabetes.

Dr. Digby Leigh wrote graphically, but more formally than in his letter to Dr. Necker, to the American Society of Anesthesiologists about the developments in Montreal. His letter was reproduced in the *ASA Newsletter* in 1940:

---

[2] The convulsive movements described here are remarkably similar to those which are currently attracting attention as a neuroexcitatory phenomenon related to the intravenous induction of anæsthesia with the relatively new anæsthetic agent propofol. The possibilty that these involuntary movements relate to an effect of the anæsthetic state, rather than to the action of propofol or a specific anæsthetic agent, is raised. The original description of this case is reproduced from the 10th March, 1943 Ciba postgraduate course handout:

> The patient was a boy of 14 years, having had morphine gr.1/12 and scopolamine gr.1/300 thirty-five minutes before being given cyclopropane by to-and-fro cannister. He began to have intermittent twitchng of his arms, legs, and abdomen shortly after induction. This continued for 15 minutes. He was intubated, and face and neck were involved. Furthermore, a history of ear trouble in childhod was elicited. There were no twitchings during recovery. COMMENT: (a) This twitching was not a true convulsion. It is sometimes seen with cyclopropane. (b) Anæsthetic agents are sometimes used to control convulsions, but can also cause them.

Dear Dr. Wood,

Everything is jumping about pretty rapidly here now. Dr. Bourne and I have the opportunity of giving some sort of a course in anesthesia as you can see by the inclosed. In addition to what is listed there, there is an honourarium of $50.00 per month. We feel that we will be able to work the candidate in on some lab work under Professor Stehle, who is head of the Department of Pharmacology at McGill University.

I thought that if you had some Canadians or other men who are looking for a place to train, that you would be kind enough to turn them in our direction.

Yours truly,

M. Digby Leigh MD.

The following is Doctor Leigh's enclosure:

GRADUATE COURSE IN ANESTHESIA

A course, covering two years of theoretical and practical instruction in Anesthesia, open to graduates who have had at least one year of intern training, will be given under the direction of:

Dr. Wesley Bourne, St Mary's Hospital, Montreal

Dr. M. Digby Leigh, Children's Memorial Hospital, Montreal

The object of this course is to give a thorough training to those who wish to specialize in the rapidly expanding field of anesthesia.

One year will be spent in each of the above-named hospitals, where room and board will be provided.

The course will begin on July 1, 1940, and applications—which should be addressed to Wesley Bourne, MD, Department of Pharmacology, McGill University, Montreal, Quebec, Canada—will be received until May 31, 1940.

Thus, Wesley Bourne's teaching and organizational abilities came to the fore during wartime, making him one of the leading figures in North American anæsthesia. In 1940, he became president of the International Anesthesia Research Society for the second time; then he was elected as the incoming president-elect of the American Society of Anesthetists Inc at its 1941 meeting, the only non-American ever to receive this honour. At the end of his term of office as president, the gavel which he had used at meetings of the society throughout the year was presented to him in appreciation for his services.

The 1941 meeting of the American Society of Anesthetists Inc/American Society of Anesthesiologists took place on 30th October, in the Mount Royal Hotel, Montreal. This was the only occasion when the society met outside of the United States. The directors announced details of society membership, which would be open to anæsthetists from the United States or Canada who passed the fellowship examination set by the American Board, with dues of $10 per year, a preliminary examination fund contribution of $1 and subscription to the journal of $3. The scientific meeting was well attended, with sixty-seven members registered. These included such famous names as Drs. Paul M. Wood (New York), Virginia Apgar (New York), Ralph M. Tovell (Hartford, Connecticut) and Harry Shields (Toronto), as well as "The Great Triumvirate" of McGill anæsthetists. Local anæsthetists presented scientific papers on thoracic anæsthesia (Georges Cousineau), acidosis in anæsthesia (M. Digby Leigh) and anæsthesia services for small hospitals (Harold R. Griffith).

Wesley Bourne was asked to comment on Dr. Leigh's paper and was extremely complimentary about his colleague's presentation. He concluded by saying that we should bear in mind that while such changes represent broadly all the deleterious actions of anæsthetics, they are closely interrelated and their interpenetration simulates the great interlocking of normal vital functions. Others drew attention to controversial clinical matters: the use of controlled pulmonary ventilation for thoracic surgery, endotracheal intubation under deep cyclopropane anæsthesia to avoid inhalation of pus from abscesses (quoting a mortality of only three in thirty-three patients), anæsthesia for pneumonectomy in an infant, inflatable cuffs causing mucosal damage in the trachea and the possible advantages of intermittent inflation of the cuff, the use of silk catheters for endotracheal intubation in small children, the potential for kinking of the new Magill tubes and enquiry about experiences with the new drug, sodium pentothal. Dr. Griffith's paper on department administration in small hospitals raised considerable discussion on the scope of the anæsthetist's work and the need to become more closely allied to the hospital administrators. This very successful meeting was marred by an accident to Dr. Adolph F. Erdmann, a founding member, who sustained a fractured skull and shoulder when he was struck by an automobile outside the Royal Victoria Hospital. He was a patient in the hospital's Ross Pavilion for the next three weeks.

The participants at the meeting were invited to visit the local Montreal hospitals to watch routine anæsthesia. This may well have been the time that Dr. Richard H. Barrett of New Hampshire wrote about when he offered these recollections of an encounter with Wesley Bourne in the early 1940s, in a letter to Dr. Charles C. Tandy. W.L.M. Chairman, dated 1st February, 1977:

> ....The only other "feat", at which I was a close observer at about that time, was watching Wesley Bourne doing full-mouth dental extractions in a dentist's office in Montreal.
>
> I entered the dentist's office with 'Wes' at 8.00 am—having walked up a long flight of rickety stairs! At a little after 9.30 am we left the office—my having observed six (6!) full-mouth extractions with immediate dentures and 'Wes' with thirty dollars ($30) in his pocket for his part of the procedures. Each patient handed Dr. Bourne five dollars, before they were anesthetized (with only nitrous oxide and oxygen). Each patient sat upright in the dental chair and the dentist lost no time in his part of the work.
>
> The patients—or victims—concerned ranged in age from 14 to 55—male and female.
>
> Following each procedure each patient walked, albeit a bit wobbly and with friendly aid, down that long flight of rickety stairs and, I suppose, out into the October air. This latter of which must have had a pleasing effect!
>
> One of the patients, who was to be 'next', was sitting not more than four feet from the dental chair observing everything which she was about to enjoy (?) And this patient was only 14 years old!
>
> Strange as it may seem, everything went smoothly; there were no tears, no crying out and no struggling on the part of the patients. It was nitrous-oxide anesthesia at its best!
>
> Incidentally—added to the festivities, about half way through this morning's list, a man, obviously a custodian of sorts, came walking through the office carrying two large buckets of garbage, apparently collected from some appartments located on the same floor as the dental office. These he carried out a back door onto the porch and dumped some of the containers (I think) below. He returned from this duty, stopped for a few minutes "to see what Doc was doing this morning" and continued on with his other duties—I guess.
>
> "Mysterious Waters to Cross"—for sure! But I am also sure that all of us have a bit of garbage in our lives somewhere.
>
> ....Wesley Bourne contributed much to the specialty of

anesthesiology—far more, probably, than will ever be known.

Please excuse my ramblings, but I thought these events might be of interest to you, and possibly, others.

Sincerely — Dick Barrett.

Dr. C.R. Stephen, one of the first wartime trainees and now active in retirement in St. Louis, Missouri, acknowledges that his career was completely changed by his attendance at the short course on anæsthesia given at McGill. He was amongst a small group of medical officers in the Royal Canadian Army Medical Corps who were sent to Montreal in November 1942 for this purpose. Wesley Bourne (consultant to the Army) led "The Great Triumvirate" in a characteristically dynamic style: finger pointing and gesticulating while he taught, gently and mesmerizingly dispelling his patients' fears of anæsthesia. The car-rides between hospitals, with Wesley Bourne in the driver's seat, invited comparison with the plight of the tuberculous patients:

> Wesley drove each of us on several occasions to the Grace Dart tuberculosis hospital to administer high spinal anæsthesia (hypobaric nupercaine) to cadaverous-looking patients for thoracoplasties. This unique and usually terrifying experience, which reminded one of the "valley of the shadow of death," was matched by the drive to and from the hospital. For Wesley liked to instruct while he drove, and when he talked he always looks at his audience, occasionally speeding through red traffic lights while he pressed his point. The result was sheer panic, with catecholamine secretions reaching pheochromocytoma-like levels. It was truly an ordeal by fire.
>
> (Stephen CR. *AHA Newsletter* 1987;5:1,11.)

He had quite a different style and personality from that of his close colleague, Dr. Harold R. Griffith (consultant to the Air Force), the chief of anæsthesia at the Homeopathic Hospital (now the Queen Elizabeth). Dr. Stephen's description of the latter cannot be bettered:

> "Uncle" Harold as we called him when he was out of earshot (he was a little deaf anyway), was much like a mother hen, quiet, serious, but with a wry wit, and such a competent anæsthetist. To watch him give a cyclopropane anesthetic was a lesson in artistic endeavor. He never appeared to worry about explosions, even though in winter the air outside was cold and dry, the operating room

windows faced the northwest, and the air inside was likewise so dry that sparks flew with gay abandon.

This sojourn in Montreal was timely and stimulating: it was the early days of "Intocostrin," the impure form of curare introduced into clinical use by Harold Griffith only months earlier, on 23rd January, 1942. There was also improvisation for anæsthetic apparatus, including the use of special large-bore urethral catheters as endotracheal tubes. The third member of the group of three was the youngest, Dr. Morton Digby Leigh (consultant to the Air Force), who was characterized by Dr. Stephen as:

> Intelligent, driven, rambunctious, a great teacher, Digby was one of the founders of pediatric anesthesia on this continent. He was the live wire of the Children's Memorial Hospital nestled on the slopes of Mount Royal in Montreal ......he pointed, cajoled and manoeuvred the student into observing the alterations associated with increasing depth of anesthesia, upper respiratory obstruction, advantages of the oral airway, intricacies of endotracheal intubation and so on.

Dr. Stephen's impressions are typical of many who came under Wesley Bourne's influence in those exciting pioneering days of modern anæsthesia and then found themselves embroiled in developing anæsthesia as a specialty. Yet, Wesley Bourne remains an enigma. He was also a philosopher and thought deeply about anæsthesia in war circumstances, the title of a paper that he read to the annual meeting of the Massachusetts Medical Society on 22nd May, 1941. He conjectured:

> Like events to those which occasioned the Peloponnesian War, though varying in force and form with every new combination of circumstances, are bound to occur as long as the nature of man continues the same.....It may be that when this has spent itself, peace will be made permanent. In the meantime, however, we must meet the vicissitudes of the hour.

Wesley Bourne and one of his colleagues from the Department of Pharmacology, Dr. N.B. Dreyer had worked closely together on the physiological effects of avertin and sodium amytal and had published several papers together in the early 1930s. Dr. Dreyer was born in South Africa and had come to Canada from England. He spent only a year at McGill between appointments to the Dalhousie faculty and had moved on to work with a pharmaceutical company in Chicago. In the *Montreal Star* on 21st May, 1941 Wesely Bourne read that Dr. Dreyer was the Canadian listed as one of the passengers on the Egyptian liner, *Zamzam,* which was en route for South Africa when it entered German occupied territory and was captured. He was interned, but there is no record of his eventual fate.

Notwithstanding the exigencies of wartime, Wesley Bourne continued to be a presence at major meetings. His presidential address to the American Society of Anesthesiologists Inc in New York on 12th February, 1942 was a passionate plea for improving the teaching of anæsthesia and its application in wartime circumstances. True to this belief, he frequently argued for keeping the principles of good anæsthetic practice, while accepting the responsibility to seek the best means of its delivery in battle conditions. He was particulary astute in his understanding of the physiological consequences of shock, and urged that the timing of morphine administration to relieve pain and anxiety should be carefully weighed against the need to resuscitate the patient. In many situations, he advocated the use of local anæsthesia as a safer choice than general anæsthesia, and the use of oxygen therapy as long as respiratory or circulatory depression continued. Typically, his meticulous approach to the delivery of care to the wounded was tempered by his search for knowledge: he asked that all records should be kept in a standard manner, so that invaluable information should not be lost.

Wesley Bourne was one of the contributing foreign editors to *Anesthesiology* when it began publication in 1940, but he never more than dabbled in editorial circles. However, his publications record did not flag during this period, although his original research reports gave way to more philosophical topics. In writing his memorial address to Francis Hoeffer McMechan, an apotheosis, he drew on Plato's philosophies, Longfellow's *A Psalm of Life,* and *The Book of Corinthians* for inspiration. Sometimes, his rhetoric and verbosity became perplexing: a dissertation on the organization of anæsthesia services is introduced in this way:

> Although in the truly etymological sense anæsthetic and æsthetic are antithetic, and it may seem paradoxical to speak of them in the same breath, yet there is much of the one in the other and æsthetic tendencies are not uncommon to anesthesia.
>
> (*Curr Res Anesth Analg* 1940;19:181-3)

His titles became magnetic. Would it be possible to ignore *De officiis in Anæsthesia,* with its prescription for the duties of an anæsthetist? The otherwise mundane is couched:

> I humbly offer my observations as sensibles in Dark Knowledge, in Way of Opinion, upon a likely interpretation of duty in anæsthesia, since that science, called Ethic, implies a sense of the responsible OUGHT in man. The many duties prescribed for anæsthesia are consecutive and interdependent. From the entire concatenation of them, in careful perspective, I should like to emphasize the advantages to be drived from the assiduous dissemination of knowledge concerning anæsthesia.
>
> (*The Journal of the Michigan State Medical Society* 1942;41:129-34)

A number of important initiatives took place despite the distractions of war. Pharmaceutical industries became aware of changing needs in anæsthesia. One prominent company, E.R. Squibb and Sons, realized that drugs needed to be stored in a suitable and reliable manner. They produced cloth-enmeshed chloroform ampoules which proved to be ideal for anæsthetizing the injured before they developed shock if they were trapped and could not be extricated promptly from their tanks. Local anæsthetics were made more useful when new topical applications, Intracaine in oil or as an ointment, became available. Single dose hypodermic units, "syrettes," provided a means of injecting drugs in an emergency and were used to administer morphine at Pearl Harbour. The introduction of curare into anæsthesia and the collaborative efforts of explorers, and the chemists and industry needed to purify and assay a compound suitable for widespread clinical use, also belongs to Montreal anæsthetists. The credit for this landmark event has gone to Harold Griffith, but the ambience in which he was working was created by Wesley Bourne. This revolutionary step in anæsthesia may have depended on the presence of all three members of "The Great Triumvirate."

In 1942, there were indications that some sort of state medicine would be introduced in Canada in the foreseeable future, and Wesley Bourne was appointed by the Canadian Medical Association to chair a committee to decide the qualifications necessary for specialist recognition in anæsthesia. Attention would be paid to experience, in terms of years spent giving anæsthesia, the percentage of a physician's income which was derived from anæsthesia and success in obtaining the Diploma in Anæsthetics of the Royal College of

Surgeons, London, England. Following approval of anæsthesia for specialist certification, it became obvious that a national specialist organization to negotiate for anæsthetists was needed. Thus, in 1943, Wesley Bourne was pivotal to the organization of the Canadian Anæsthetists' Society (CAS), fifteen years after he had witnessed the demise of the original Canadian Society of Anæsthetists (CSA).

The CAS adopted the seal and motto which Wesley Bourne had designed for the CSA, with the help of the artist, A. Sherriff Scott, two decades earlier. This was the only thing which was common to both of these societies. The same motto in Greek "We watch closely those who sleep" was retained below the seal and the words "Canadian Society of Anæsthetists. Incorporated 1920" which encircled the seal, became "Canadian Anæsthetists' Society." Although its symbolism has been explained on the basis of the analogy of the Cave of Hypnos with anæsthesia; a broader interpretation, based on a deeper understanding of Wesley Bourne, invites consideration. He read and quoted often from Plato's *Republic*,[3] frequently writing about the likeness of anæsthesia to the ideal society for which Plato aimed. This "just" society was based on Socrates' code of ethics, which he had taught to his student, Plato, and in which there would be equal justice for the individual and society. Education would be provided only by the state and the Academy would provide courses to educate people. Philosophers would govern this ideal state. The philosophical and religious elements embraced by this society are discussed in a series of related similes: the Sun, the Divided Line and the Cave. These use the freeing of prisoners from the dark cave to show how man moves from illusion to philosophy; seeing the light of the sun as "the vision of the form of the good." Once released, the prisoners achieve the supreme vision and are obliged to share it with the other prisoners, but are unwilling to return to the darkness of the cave.

If the Cave of Hypnos of the CAS seal is likened to the cave of Plato's simile, then a deeper significance may be sought and a wider interpretation of its meaning offered. The key fact is that Hypnos is depicted outside, rather than inside, his mythical home. This draws an analogy with the contemporaneous state of the development of the specialty of anæsthesia in the 1920s and 1940s.

---

[3] Plato's *Republic* was written around 375 BC as a philosophical dialogue on "What is justice?" between Socrates and Plato's older brothers, Glaucon and Adeimantus.

Plato taught that the average man knows the difference between substance and shadow in the physical sense, but his moral and intellectual opinions bear little on the real truth. Only philosophical leadership can produce the organized society in which true justice is found.

Surely the specialty of anæsthesia, represented by Hypnos, had emerged from the cave of darkness as scientific understanding of anæsthesia dawned. The formation of the CSA and CAS, would be seen by Wesley Bourne as the formation of such an ideal professional society; led by the academic "philosophers", who had just emerged into the "light" of their science. Their struggles to organize the society of anæsthetists, while providing education and service to others, would be no less than those difficulties overcome by the philosophers who achieved the supreme vision of Plato's Cave.

All the while, Bourne's interest in good literature never flagged and he managed to find time for a considerable amount of recreational reading. The future wife of his son Douglas, who was of Finnish origin, read works by Jane Austen, Charlotte Brontë and Charles Dickens as a result of his influence. He still found time for his family and when Hilary Bourne, his nephew, arrived in Montreal to begin his medical studies at McGill, he was met by Wesley Bourne at the train station and taken to his home on Holton Avenue in Westmount to stay until he found suitable lodging near the university. Hilary says that he immediately noticed that Wesley Bourne's energy and enthusiasm had not changed in the twelve years since they last met. He had tremendous drive and was, perhaps, a little reckless at times. In that first Fall he drove Hilary in his 1938 V-8 Ford to St. Marguerite, in the Laurentians, to show him the magnificence of the colours of the maple trees. On the way there he was bubbling with chatter, pointing out things of interest along the way. At one point Hilary glanced at the speedometer and discovered that it read 95 mph, a speed at which he had never travelled before, or since. He tells this story to conjure up a picture of Wesley Bourne, the man; a man who was always in over-drive.

The founding of the Department of Anesthesia at McGill was the culmination of Bourne's wartime achievements. During the war, anæsthesia had become relevant to contemporary needs. Teaching programmes had been started and clinical service requirements addressed. The scientific basis of anæsthesia was appreciated in Canada almost entirely as a result of Bourne's efforts. The earliest remaining record of the founding of the department is in a letter from McGill's Principal and Vice-Chancellor, F. Cyril James, to Wesley Bourne:

written on 15th November, 1945 when Bourne was still an unpaid Lecturer in the Department of Pharmacology. The date on which the establishment of the new Department of Anæsthesia was formally recognized appears to have been delayed until the next year, 1946. Regardless of which inaugural date you choose, or whether confusion has been introduced by a secretarial error in the recorded dates, it is undisputed that Wesley Bourne founded the first autonomous department of anæsthesia in Canada at McGill.

V

FOUNDING THE MCGILL DEPARTMENT (1945-50)

McGill found itself in an evolving multicultural milieu, within a city which increasingly acnowledged "the French fact." Pierre Elliot Trudeau had graduated from the Université de Montréal during a period of student unrest. The English and French communities in the city were making tentative alliances and McGill established a French summer school as a gesture towards the promotion of bilingualism. Only a few minor scandals tarnished the image of McGill: espionage charges were laid against a member of the Chemistry Department, thought to be associated with a Russian cypher clerk in Ottawa. However, these were more than off-set by recognition of the wartime contributions to the atomic bomb programme and chemical warfare by Otto Maass, the head of the Chemistry Department, which encouraged the expansion in post-war research.

Returning veterans swelled the student body to 8,237 by 1947; fifty percent larger than its pre-war size. This unprecedented increase in numbers created the necessity of coping with their needs and permanently changed the character of the University. Buildings on campus were extended and upgraded, but fell short of requirements. Accommodation had to be found quickly. Consequently, twenty miles away Sir William Dawson College opened, occupying a former air training school. About $40 million was needed, but private donations raised only $7 million towards the total, forcing the University administration to turn towards the government for funding. The financial crisis would become as much a part of the University's history during the first two decades of peacetime as the major technological developments stimulated by the war. The explosion of scientific knowledge and zeal for teaching, which characterized the period, percolated into all disciplines. Therefore, the decision of the Principal and the Board of Governors of the University to establish the Department of Anesthesia from 1st September, 1945 was a logical extension, and culmination, of Wesley Bourne's wartime efforts. This was the pivotal step towards the recognition of anæsthesia as a specialty in Canada, as well as a tribute to Wesley Bourne's personal achievements.

There were no other independent university departments of anæsthesia in Canada at that time, although they existed in the United States at Madison, Wisconsin (Ralph Waters, 1933), Columbus, NY (D.A. Rovenstine, 1938), Harvard, Boston (Henry K. Beecher, first North American endowed Chair of Anæsthesia, 1941) and Oxford, England (Robert Macintosh, Nuffield Chair, the first endowed chair in anæsthesia, 1937). In Canada, the appointments of Drs. Webster in Winnipeg (1905) and Johnston in Toronto (1907) as university lecturers in anæsthesia had been made within their respective departments of medicine and surgery. The first autonomous department of anæsthesia in Canada was created with Wesley Bourne's appointment as chairman of the McGill Department of Anesthesia in 1945. With the approval of Dr. J. Meakins, the Dean of Medicine; F. Cyril James, the Principal and Vice-Chancellor, informed Wesley Bourne by letter of 15th November, 1945:

> Dear Dr. Bourne,
>
> I am very glad indeed to tell you that the Board of Governors at its meeting yesterday afternoon appointed you to be Chairman of the newly created Department of Anæsthesia for the current academic session, ending on May 31st next.
>
> I know how deeply interested you have been in the creation of this department and in the program of work you expect to carry out. I should like, therefore, to offer my warm good wishes to you as you take the helm for this first section of its course.
>
> Cordially yours,

Thus, Wesley Bourne was appointed for the balance of the 1945-6 academic year, with the commencement of his chairmanship retroactive to 1st September, 1945, according to his staff records. A brief report was made in the Montreal *Gazette* on the day following the Board of Governors' meeting. However, formal release of the news of the establishment of the Department of Anæsthesia within the Faculty of Medicine at McGill, under the chairmanship of Wesley Bourne, appeared first in the *Montreal Star* on 31st January, 1946. This announcement claimed that "the news was disclosed today and had been delayed until the organization of the new department was well underway." The "University Notes" section of the *Canadian Medical Association Journal* carried a notification in March 1946 and this was soon followed by exposure to a wider audience in the *British Journal of Anæsthesia* and the *American Society of Anesthesiologists* Newsletter[1].

The wartime programme of teaching provided McGill the model for

---

[1] "University Notes. McGill University." *Can Med Assoc J* 1946;54:300. Followed by: *Br J Anæsth* 1946-7;20:105 and the *ASA Newsletter*. March 1946, no.3:1.

training specialists in anæsthesia. This has remained almost unchanged for the last fifty years, despite the succession of chairmen, faculty and residents who have passed through the system. The McGill diploma course in anæsthesia was soon instituted as a three-year basic science programme (given by Professors K.I. Melville, D.L. Thompson, H.E. Hoff and C.P. Martin, all of whom had been associated with Wesley Bourne in the laboratories), combined with a series of weekly teaching rounds given by anæsthetists (Drs. Ron Stephen, Harry Slater, W. Cullen, André Pasquet, Romeo Rochette and Dick Gilbert and others). Clinical work was undertaken in the English and French hospitals in Montreal. Once a week, on Monday evenings, French and English anæsthetists (staff, residents and visitors) congregated in the Ciba building to discuss interesting cases, show films, demonstrate hypnosis or debate topics in anæsthesia. Dr. Ron Stephen, by then secretary of the Canadian Anæsthetists' Society, began to announce the weekly meetings, with a list of topics, as a regular feature in the *American Society of Anesthesiologists Newsletter* from October 1949.

The first eight anæsthetists who graduated from the three-year postgraduate course in anæsthesia, with the award of a diploma in anæsthesia from McGill, were featured in an article in the *Montreal Daily Star* on Saturday, 29th May, 1948. The rigorous nature of their training was noted and compared favourably with the shorter two-year fellowship programme required by the American Board of Anesthesiology and the Royal College of Physicians and Surgeons of Canada. Seven were veterans and one was a civilian doctor. They had all accepted appointments in North American cities and would go on to train anæsthetists in those centres. They were listed as Drs. R.E.H. Farquharson (Edmonton, intending to return there), H.A. Kester (London, Ontario, moving to San Francisco), F.W. McCaffrey (Montreal, returning to the army), D.H. McIntyre (Edmonton, moving to Vancouver), A. Pasquet (Montreal, with a staff position at the Montreal Neurological Institute), H.M. Slater (Toronto, becoming assistant anæsthetist at Montreal Children's Hospital), W.E. Upthegrove (Toronto, going to the University of Saskatchewan) and E. Webb (Stratford, Ontario, moving to a staff anæsthetist position at Vancouver General Hospital). Three of these anæsthetists, Drs. Kester, McCaffrey and Webb, are now living in retirement in the Vancouver, BC region. Dr. Frank W. McCaffrey wrote in December 1995, to say that he owes most of his professional life to Wesley Bourne, for the following reasons:

> Upon my return from overseas duties with the RCAMC in WW2, I

asked for a temporary posting to the Quebec Military Hospital (the district in which I had enlisted). I had become interested in Anæsthesia (almost accidentally Overseas....a story in itself!)

In those days, there were only 3-4 places in Canada where one could go for anæsthesia training. The two best ones were McGill in Montreal, and Toronto's Faculty of Medicine Specialization Course. After spending a short while at home, I took a trip to Montreal to be interviewed by the Department of Anæsthesia Head at McGill. This turned out to be Professor Wesley Bourne, a genius-at-organization type of man, who had then developed and established the McGill Diploma Course in Anæsthesiology. We had a very long talk indeed! I told him that I had gained some experience in anæsthesia Overseas, and at that point it was my intention to go into general practice somewhere in a smaller community. I wanted further instruction and experience in anæsthesia for children, women, and older people, with whom I had no experience at all....Well, Wesley Bourne turned out to be a "super salesman!".....He pointed out to me the rapid advances now taking place in Anæsthesiology....that I should forget this part-time stuff, and instead, enroll in his new Diploma Course!...I pointed out that I was still in the Army, was in effect recently married, and could not take take on this Course, and at the same time meeting our living responsibilities.... After much talking and thinking, he asked me, if he could possibly arrange things with the Army to subsidize me, would I then be willing to consider joining his course to become a full-fledged specialist in Anæsthesiology!....I doubted that this could be done that easily....but in a very little time, Dr. Bourne arranged for me to be transferred to the then Montreal Military Hospital (which soon after became a combined Veterans Hospital, and subsequently became known as Queen Elizabeth Hospital, if I remember correctly)....There I functioned as a Resident in Anæsthesia, while continuing to hold my Army rank and pay, such as it was!.....Dr. Bourne then arranged subsequently for me to rotate residencies in the University teaching hospitals which were participating in the McGill training programs. When I was rotated to another hospital, Dr. Bourne would post one of his other Residents to Queen Elizabeth Hospital, "doing my duties." Dr. Bourne had meanwhile given me credits for the experience gained Overseas.

In this manner, I rotated through the various anæsthesia residencies of McGill's Teaching Hospitals, receiving all round good training. I opted for an extra six months because it was an opportunity to work at the Children's Hospital, although Dr. Bourne had given me credit of one year for Army experience[2].

Along with Drs......I graduated in McGill's first full diploma Course in Anæsthesiology. So, you see, I do owe a great deal to Wesley Bourne!

Sincerely, Frank W McCaffrey MD FRCP[3]

Before 1939, qualified physicians could claim to be "specialists" in the field in which they practised, but a more precise definition of a specialist was needed, in part as a basis for negotiating appropriate remuneration. Discussions began on the requirements for specialist certification and in 1942, certification in anæsthesia was granted by the Royal College of Physicians and Surgeons of Canada, although anæsthetists were still excluded from becoming fellows of the College. The first examination for specialist certificates of the Royal College of Physicians and Surgeons of Canada was held in 1946 and for fellowships, modified for individual specialties, in 1947.

Wesley Bourne became a fellow of the Faculty of Anæsthetists of Great Britain and Ireland (FFARCS) in 1946. He was in a list of internationally renowned anæsthetists, including T. Cecil Gray, C. Langton Hewer, E.A. Pask, Ralph M. Waters and Geoffrey Kaye, who were elected to the fellowship during the first year that it was established[4]. Since he held a fellowship in medicine, Wesley Bourne was the only anæsthetist granted entry to full fellowship before 1951. He was selected to serve on the Montreal sub-committee of the Royal College which drafted the regulations for the essential requirements for graduate training in 1948 and formulated guidelines for admissibilty to examination and

---

[2] In the British army, the opportunity to complete specialist anæsthesia training, which required at least six months release from the army, was not achieved by members of the RAMC until 1968.

[3] Dr. Frank McCaffrey now lives in White Rock BC. In his memorabilia he found the newspaper clip from the *Montreal Daily Star* and pictures of Kester Brown, himself and Wesley Bourne in academic dress at graduation. He believes that a number of those first graduates, including Dr. Slater, are now deceased.

[4] The Faculty of Anæsthetists. *Br J Anæsth* 1948-9;21:154.

standards for hospitals approved for teaching. Entry to full fellowship in anæsthesia in Canada was delayed until 1951, but its introduction aggravated divisions between anæsthetists by resulting in a dual professional standard of certificate and fellowship recognition. This situation lasted for twenty years until 1971, when certification was discontinued and a single standard of fellowship was introduced, belatedly giving anæsthetists the same status as other medical specialties in the country.

Wesley Bourne rose quickly up the academic ladder. He was promoted to part-time assistant professor in September, 1946, at an annual salary of $125, associate professor in 1948 with an increase in salary to $175, then professor in June, 1949. To integrate research formally into the strong clinical anæsthetic department, he actively recruited associates with research interests, including Dr. E.A. Pask from England, who spent a year at the Montreal Neurological Institute[5]. Along the way, valuable colleagues were lost; notably Dr. M. Digby Leigh who moved to British Columbia as director of anæsthesia at Vancouver General Hospital in 1947, although he was soon replaced by the equally formidable Dr. Ron Stephen as director of the Montreal Children's Hospital department. Frank recollections of Dr. Dick Gilbert, from England, underscore other realities of recruitment into the department after 1945:

> So we immigrated and I arrived in Montreal and I went to call on Wesley Bourne. He was away. I was told at the Vic that they had no room for any more anæsthetists. Moreover, I was told that they did not want any British graduates there..........I made other enquiries and I was told that if I applied to Toronto and went there, I would probably have my throat cut because they did not want an invasion of British ex-army anæsthetists or British graduates to come over here. They were very serious about that.......I met Fraser Gurd Sr., who had just taken over a little hospital called the Women's General Hospital, which is now the Reddy. It had got into rather ill odour

[5] Dr. Edgar Pask had made ground-breaking and convincing contributions with his research in England. During the war he allowed himself to be anæsthetized and thrown into a swimming pool to test the efficacy of the Mae West survival vest. He also volunteered for simulated high altitude flight testing in which he breathed hypoxic, 7% oxygen mixtures. The story is told that he needed a subject to show that regional anæsthesia could be induced electrically, so he applied an electric current across his leg, made an incision and sutured the wound painlessly, only to discover that the apparatus was not plugged into the electric socket!

> because of a reputation for doing abortions, so he cleared out the staff and put in three young men, a pathologist, a radiologist and myself, as a whole time anæsthetist, paid by the hospital.

Dr. Gilbert completed his examinations to practise in North America and in 1949 Wesley Bourne, who had become his mentor, appointed him as a lecturer at McGill. Dick Gilbert never forgot those legendary drives to and from the Grace Dart Hospital. Bourne insisted on driving and when Gilbert said "I want to stop to mail a letter," he replied "I can mail a letter without getting out of the car." Bourne reached out of the car and put the letter in the mail box, but forgot that the car was on a hill and he jammed his arm between the mail box and the car. His language was awful. Gilbert knew both Wesley Bourne and Harold Griffith well and made the astute observation "Wesley promoted Harold because he was a good organizer and he was respected by everyone....as a pair, Wesley made the bullets and Harold fired them..." In time, Dr. Gilbert would follow both of these men in the chairmanship of the department.

The 100th anniversary of William Thomas Green Morton's first public demonstration of ether in Boston on 16th October, 1846[6] in the Massachusetts General Hospital, Boston, was approaching. To mark the anniversary, Professor H.K. Beecher, professor of surgery in Boston, was invited to visit Montreal before the celebrations in Boston. He lectured to students in the Diploma Course in Anæsthesia and to medical students at McGill and the University of Montreal. After visiting the French and English hospitals, he was the speaker at the evening meeting in the Ciba building: much as the visiting professor programme works today. Centennial commemorations took place in London, England from 30th October to 1st November, 1946. Wesley Bourne was invited to take part in the celebrations by the Association of Anæsthetists of Great Britain and Ireland and he went there as a representative for both Canada and the United States. Under the existing university regulations, he could only be reimbursed for a "railroad and pullman" fare to Boston (as he was delivering a paper at a scientific gathering) for the "Centenary of Morton's Demonstration of the Use of Ether" on 15th to 17th October, but the Board of Governors declined to contribute to the cost of Wesley Bourne's trip to England. He flew to England in a converted Lancaster bomber, describing a sensation of vibration that lasted for two or three days after he landed.

---

[6] Morton had administered ether in his dental office since 30th September or 1st October 1846.

"The Centennium of Anæsthesia," a paper written in Wesley Bourne's philosophical style, describes that first administration of ether and recognizes famous men of the same period; Henry Longfellow (1807-1882), Louis Pasteur (1822-1895), Charles Darwin (1809-1882), Victor Hugo (1802-1885), John Ruskin (1819-1900) and many others. Experiences at these successful conferences in Boston and England are recorded in two parts in *Anesthesiology* in 1948. Bourne describes watching Dr. (later, Sir) Geoffrey Organe working at the Westminster Hospital in London and meeting the retired Sir Francis Shipway for lunch. He also recounts a reception at Canada House and then a trip to Cambridge to visit Charles Bourne, his nephew who was studying law. He enjoyed seeing the countryside and toured Lichfield Cathedral. Before proceeding to Ireland he visited Shropshire, the birthplace of Henry Hill Hickman (1800-1830) of carbon dioxide suspended animation fame and William Withering (1741-1799) known for the introduction of digitalis as a therapeutic agent. He returned to Liverpool and Oxford, where he was hosted by Robert Macintosh, before leaving for home.

A few days after arriving in Montreal he received a letter from Dr. Georges Cousineau. Wesley Bourne admitted that it caused his eyes to fill with tears:

> Bywater 1042
> 3600 Blvd Gouin ouest
> Montreal
>
> Docteur Wesley Bourne
> Montreal
>
> Cher Docteur
>
> A notre dernière réunion de la section Québecoise de la Société Canadienne d'Anesthésie, il est proposé et adopté à l'unanimité qu'un vote de remerciement soit addressé au docteur Wesley Bourne qu'a bien voulu aller nous représenter à l'occasion de la célébration du Centenaire de la découverte de l'éther. A cette occasion, spontanément tous les membres présent détient les cordons de leur bourse et vous offre, mon cher Docteur, l'expression tangible de leur reconnaissance et me charge de vous remettre le chèque ci-inclus.
>
> Veuillez, cher confrère aîné, accepter ce modeste cadeau de vos amis sincères, les Anesthésistes de Quebec. Nous sommes fiers, nous

sommes reconnaissants et nous voulons suivre toujours (c'est à vous maintenant que nous appliquons cette expression que vous appliquez autrefois au Docteur Laroque) notre "panache blanc."

Sincèrement,
Georges Cousineau
29 Novembre 1946

When Wesley Bourne's account of his visit to the ether centennial celebrations was published in *Anesthesiology* in May and July, 1948, Wesley Bourne sent reprints to his colleague and wrote on them in his own hand: "Un grand homme d'anesthésie, Georges Cousineau. Tous allèrent faire compliments à mes sentiments les meilleurs, Wesley Bourne." and "to Georges Cousineau, with compliments and deep affection from Wesley." Cousineau was a graduate of the Université de Montréal and worked with Bethune on thoracic surgical cases. He was the first anæsthetist to introduce intravenous anæsthesia into Canada, using hexobarbitone obtained from Germany by Bethune. Harold Griffith showed him intubating techniques and Wesley Bourne and he were active in several of the same societies. Cousineau began a residency programme for French Quebec anæsthetists. The interactions amongst this group, Bourne, Griffith and Cousineau, promoted collegiality between English and French speaking anæsthetists.

International liaisons were not always as satisfactory as Wesley Bourne's centennial visit to Boston and England. In 1949 Bourne was the Canadian delegate to the Latin-American Congress of Anesthesiology in Buenos Aires, the inaugural meeting of the Brazilian Society of Anesthesiology. Dr. Edward B. Tuohy of the Mayo clinic, Rochester, Minnesota, represented the United States and an announcement to this effect appeared in the *American Society of Anesthesiologists Newsletter*. Subsequently, Wesley Bourne was listed in the 1951 directory of the Cuban Society of Anesthesiologists as an honorary member, along with John Lundy of the Mayo Clinic and Robert Macintosh from Oxford, England. This directory was sent to the Australian Society of Anæsthetists to encourage its participation in the affairs of the Cuban society. However, the Australian society questioned the Cuban society's credibility, despite the powerful recommendations implied by the honorary membership list. The undertaking of this society, "to develop an effortless anesthesia machine, which changes many theories in anesthesiology," raised uncertainties, but embryonic connections were still forged. Pressures to increase Australian involvement raised suspicions and it was soon learned that the National Medical College of Cuba did not acknowledge this group; an incontrovertible reason for the Australian Society to sever relationships with the Cuban Society of Anesthesiologists.

French Canadian colleagues were some of Wesley Bourne's closest friends. Quebec anæsthetists presented him with his portrait, painted by A. Sheriff Scott, the same struggling young artist who had earlier designed the CSA emblem, in recognition of their high esteem for a distinguished confrère. Dr. Moise Clermont of Montreal, president of the Quebec division of the Canadian Anæsthetists' Society, made the presentation at the 25th joint meeting of the International Anesthesia Research Society and the International College of Anesthetists at Miami Beach, Florida in October, 1950. Wesley Bourne studied French, as well as Spanish, in his efforts to communicate more empathetically. In his fifties, he even embarked on learning Russian; at first from taped lessons, awakening his family with his repetitions at six and seven o'clock in the morning. To improve his Russian, he took private lessons from Mr. Ter Asaturoff, a white Russian, who became a close friend. He was a charming man and the family enjoyed listening to his many tales.

Wesley Bourne continued as professor and chairman until his retirement in 1950. Given his committment to the organization of teaching, international liaison, administration of a fledgling department and clinical responsibilties, it is surprising that he continued to contribute to the journals so prolifically. His writing reflected the interests of his later years. The original research of his youth was replaced by a commitment to teaching and organization, interpreted with the intense philosophical approach which characterized his maturity. Experience allowed him to be authoratative, or to reminisce on his travels abroad. He had much to impart.

From his address to the Morton Centennial, Boston:

> Nearly always innovation in anæsthesia has come from the laboratory. This time, it came from the pharmacologists, G.H.W. Lucas and V.E. Henderson, of Toronto University. In August, 1929, they reported "A new anæsthetic gas: cyclopropane."......Cyclopropane was first administered to man, in the clinical way, by Ralph M. Waters in 1930, at the University of Wisconsin..
>
> (Gaseous anæsthetics. *Anesthesiology* 1947;8:227-35)

On the three-year diploma course in anæsthesia:

> ...he who learns from many masters is bound to be more versatile and more percipient than he who ranges under one rubric (Post-graduate education in anæsthesia. *Virginia Medical Monthly* 1948;75:1-3)

Classical quotations served to enliven his view of the clinical anæsthetist. Extracting from the work of Cyrene in 400AD, writing in praise of baldness: "the balder a man is, the wiser and the more divine we may take him to be.... of all the shapes, the sphere is the most perfect—and that is the shape of the bald head." This introduces the article "At the Head of the Table" (*California Medicine* 1948;69:425-8) which describes the matrix of patient care in which the anæsthetist functions; from learning, inquiring research, to shortage of skilled anæsthetists and the like. In placing the anæsthetist at "the head of the table", Wesley Bourne borrows from Dr. H.W. Kearney, whom he might have heard speaking at the Interstate Association of Anesthetists, Cincinnati in 1915[7]. They both see the anæsthetist as being in control, not only of the conduct of anæsthesia, but as the person who integrates all the activities in the operating room. Dr. Kearney states in a practical manner, that the anæsthetist must have a viewpoint on factors which influence surgical mortality, whereas Wesley Bourne's interpretation gives the anæsthetist, ultimately, the power to see and to know and to think with understanding in the attainment of the philosophical "divine tranquilty."

Selecting the "best" from these philosophical dissertations is a test to the reader. Suffice to take just one more; "Wise indifference of the wise in anesthesia" (*Am J Obst Gyne* 1948;55:711-6). The title, "Wise Indifference of the Wise" is taken from Tennyson's poem *A Dedication.* It has an epigraph from Aristotle, in Greek, "Just as to practise medicine and healing consists not in applying or not applying the knife, in using or not using medicines, but in doing so in a certain way." This article is the transcription of an address to the Annual Meeting of the American Association of Obstetricians, Gynecologists and Abdominal Surgeons, Hot Springs, Virginia, in 1947. Essentially, it puts forward the outline of the history of anæsthesia and thoughts on its present status

---

[7] Kearney, H.W. "Surgical mortality from the standpoint of the anæsthetist." *American Journal of Surgery*, 1916;30:66-8.

following the centennary celebrations of the introduction of ether and coincident with chloroform's 100th year anniversary. However, it is illuminated by the literature, so well known to Wesley Bourne and so apt in its application:

> Mankind so far has been ruled by things and not by thought. (John Dewey)
>
> Why, who makes much of miracles?
> As to me I know of nothing else but miracles. (Walt Whitman)
>
> Bethink you too that perhaps in knowing me you know the instrument of a Purpose, the tool of a Hand too large for your sight as now to compass. (Sir Charles Sherrington)

On the toxicity of anæsthetic drugs, particularly on the liver, Wesley Bourne draws inferences:

> Thus allured ineludibly, indeed ineluctably, we find ourselves following an illimitable course crossed, it is true, by many a bourne but with never-finishing frontiers, over each of which the beacons of those beyond become more and more beckoning as one by one measures are made sure. He who would go this way, in the language of Tolstoy, must eschew the only two sources of human vice, idleness, and superstition, and pursue the only two virtues, activity and intelligence.

He couches the goals and achievements so far in anæsthesia as "bournes" which have been overcome, and finishes by stating that the "cynosures" of the anæsthetist (derived from the Greek for the constellation of Ursa Minor, to mean the attraction of the subject) are not just the physiological matters, but the education exemplified by the increasing number of postgraduate courses in anæsthesia. He opines that "Inexorably the investigator flags nor swerves from the path of discovery, while he does not allow himself to marvel immoderately. He will keep in mind the advice of Horace 'To wonder at nothing is about the one and only thing which can make a man happy, and keep him so.'"

As Wesley Bourne moved towards the close of his career, he touched many with a sermon he preached on "Hospital Sunday" on 21st May, 1950, in

Christ Church Cathedral[8] in Montreal. His title "Cultivate your Garden" concealed the true meaning, illustrated by debate of the art and science of medicine, ethics and religion. Reference to this sermon was found in the *British Journal of Anæsthesia* in Harold Griffith's tribute to Wesley Bourne in his retirement year[9] and it is included, in its entirety, in the book *Mysterious Waters to Guard,* published in Wesley Bourne's retirement. He quotes from Lord Elton's *Two Villages...* "there can in fact be no collectively good people unless there be many separate good men......Cultivez votre jardin. Cultivate your gardens! A great many tidy and fertile plots make a prosperous country. Cultivate your gardens!" Wesley Bourne translated this to his meaning "let us cultivate the garden of youth, so to tend the coming generations," echoing Dr. F.H. McMechan's prophetic quotation from *The Bridge Builder* a quarter of a century earlier:

> A youth whose feet must pass this way,
> This chasm has been as nought to me,
> To that fair-haired youth may a pitfall be:
> He too must crosss in the twilight dim -
> Good friend, I am building this bridge for him!

Retirement approached. In a letter of 6th December, 1949 F. Cyril James anticipated Wesley Bourne's departure from the McGill faculty on 31st May, 1950, forty-three years after he first entered the University. It is best to reproduce the letter in its entirety, as it underscores the profound changes in attitudes which had evolved in that time and marks, with a ring of finality, the end of this formative era in Canadian anæsthesia:

> Dear Professor Bourne,
>
> You already know that the University and the teaching Hospitals some three years ago adopted a resolution providing for the retirement of part-time members of the staff at the end of the academic session following their sixty-second birthday. That resolution, which had its origins in the proposals of the late Dr.

---

[8] Wesley's son, Douglas was not sure if this was the church, and thought it may have been the Church of St. Andrew and St. Paul. However, he and his brother John are now agreed that the sermon was delivered in Christ Church Cathedral.

[9] Griffith, H.G. "Eminent anæsthetists, no.6. Wesley Bourne." *Br J Anæsth* 1951;23:186-95.

C.K.P. Henry and others, comes into effect on August 31, 1950.

Officially, therefore, I must play the role of timekeeper, but both officially and personally I want to tell you how much I appreciate the great contribution that you have made during the years are encompassed in my own memory, so that these words of personal thanks recall to my mind the individual occasions when I have benefited from your advice and counsel, as well as those others when I have known of specific things that you had done, even though we had not talked of them.

Your formal retirement from McGill and from the staff of the Royal Victoria Hospital will not, I know, mean retirement from practice, but I hope that it may give you a little more leisure and the opportunity to do some of the pleasant things to which you have looked forward. I hope, too, that we may have many opportunities to sit down together and chat about medical education and practice.

May I add to these words of thanks my warmest good wishes for Christmastide, and remain, as always,

Cordially yours,

The Canadian Anæsthetists' Society showed its appreciation of Wesley Bourne's contribution to the specialty by naming its annual meeting in Montebello, Quebec, in 1951 in his honour. In thanking the gathering, Wesley Bourne said "Never has our position been so strong, and, if we only will realize it, we actually are able to insist that proper principles of practice be enforced." Was he having "Fun" again? Was he really reinforcing the meaning of the CSA seal of 1922, enshrined by the assembled CAS membership? Did he want the audience to read Plato once more and see that anæsthesia had indeed come out of the darkness and could control its own destiny? He went on to say "In my opinion, even more important than declarations of policy or making of rules, is the necessity for each one of us, young and old, to resolve that he will give the best kind of anæsthetics of which he is capable, without regard for when this may involve sacrifice of time and leisure or material reward." Perhaps, in this, he demonstrates his foresight. He was explaining what lay ahead for anæsthetists in achieving their ideal, as depicted in Plato's Republic.

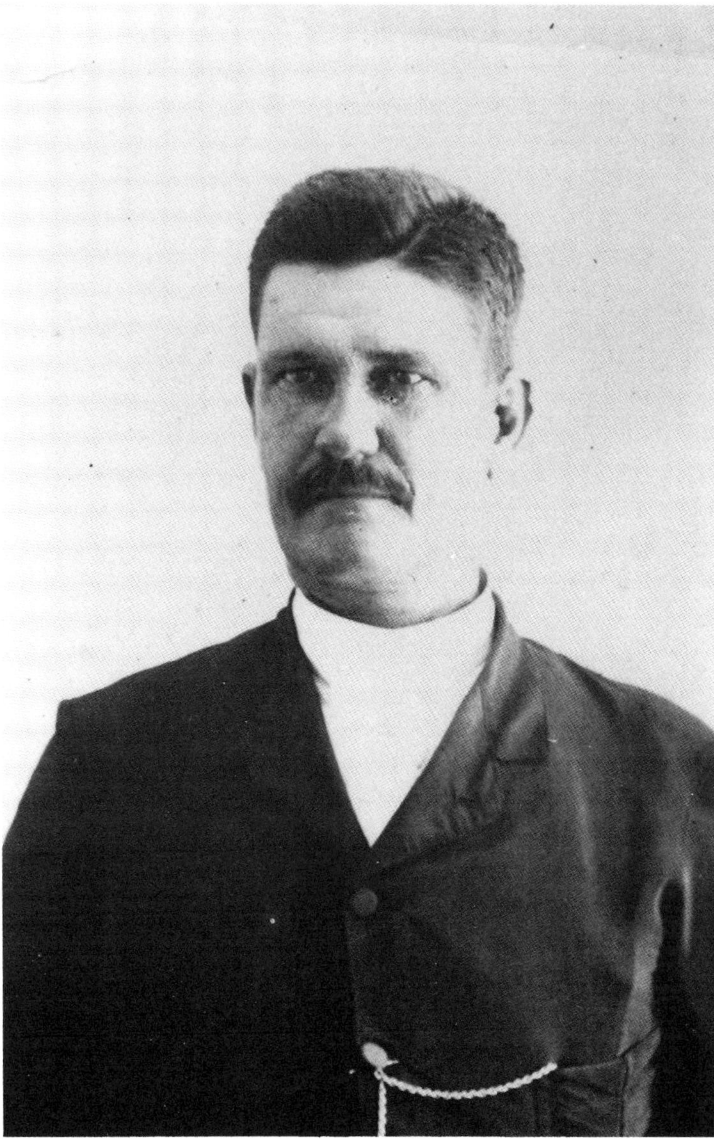

Figure 1. James Thomas Bourne (1851-1923)—Wesley Bourne's father.

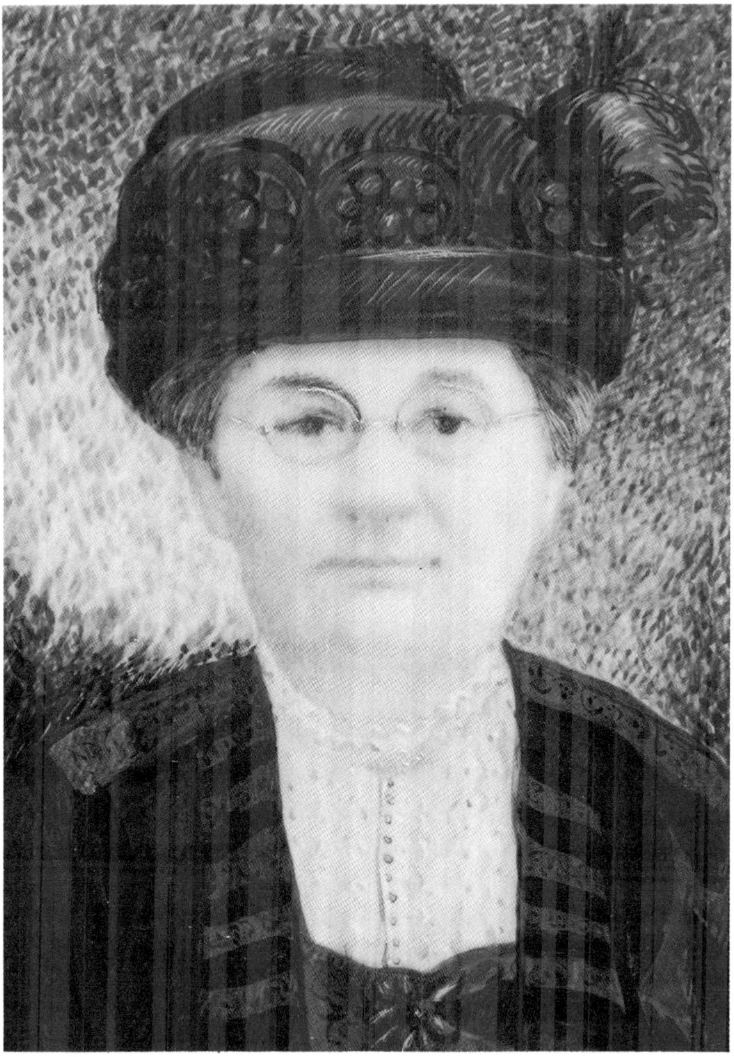

Figure 2. Mary Elizabeth (Harding) Bourne (1849-1937)—Wesley Bourne's mother.

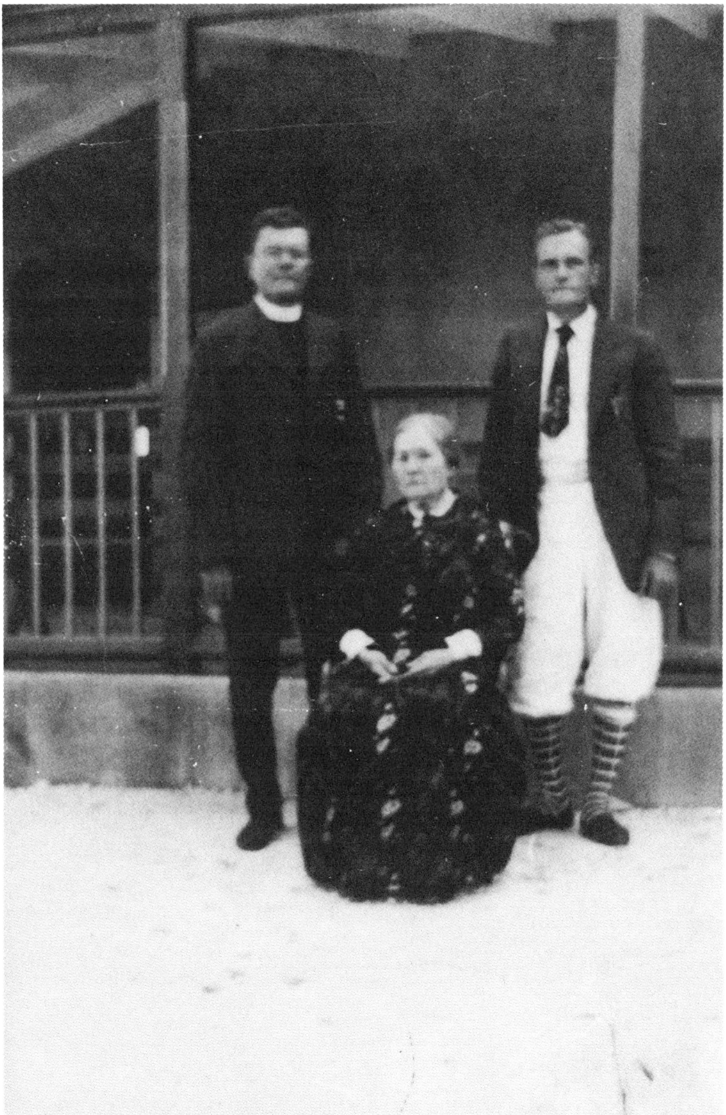

Figure 3. James and Wesley Bourne with their mother in front of "Newhaven," during a visit to Barbados in 1931.

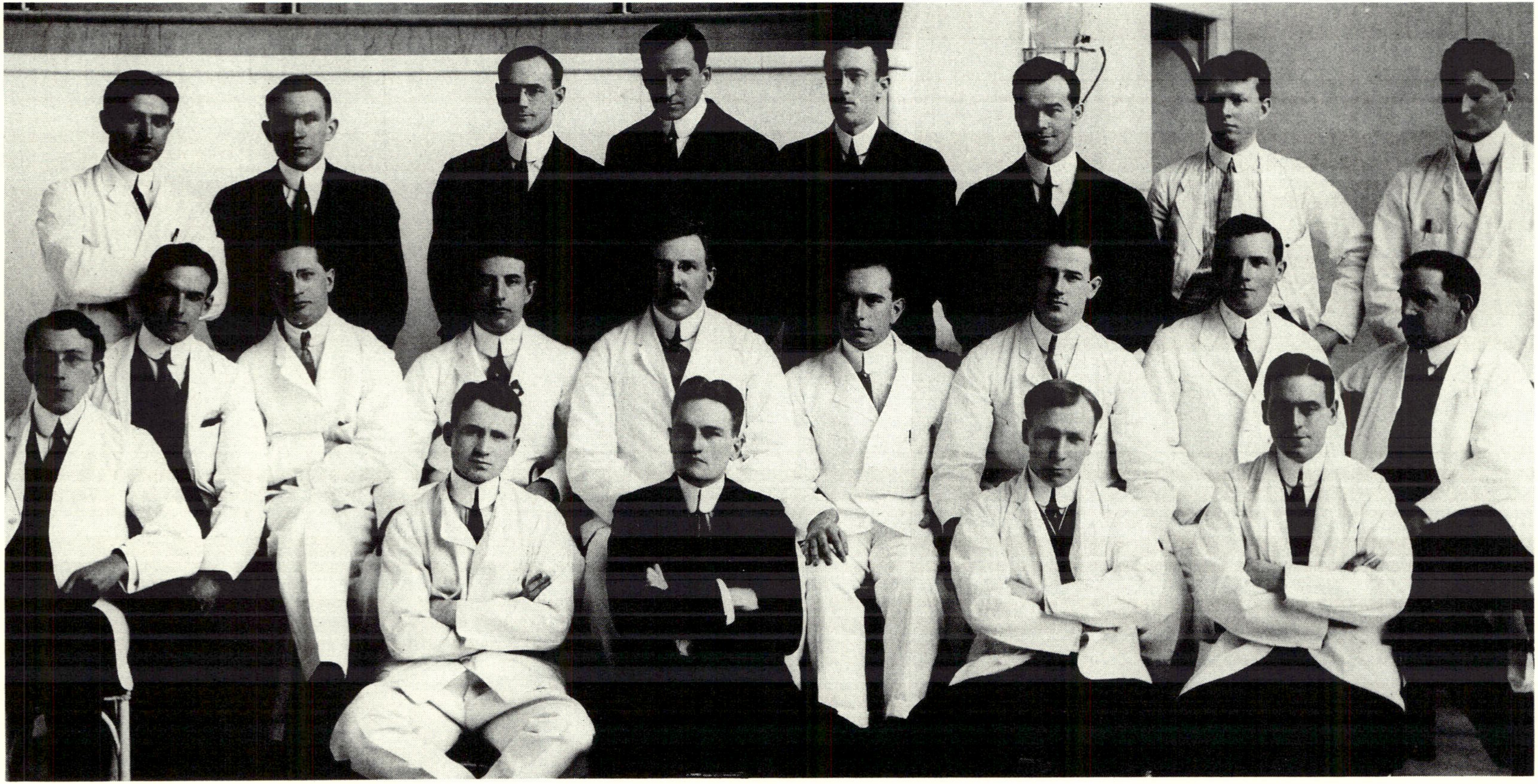

Figure 4. Royal Victoria Hospital, Montreal, Resident Staff 1912-1913. First row centre: Dr. L.W. Bourne, House Anaesthetist.

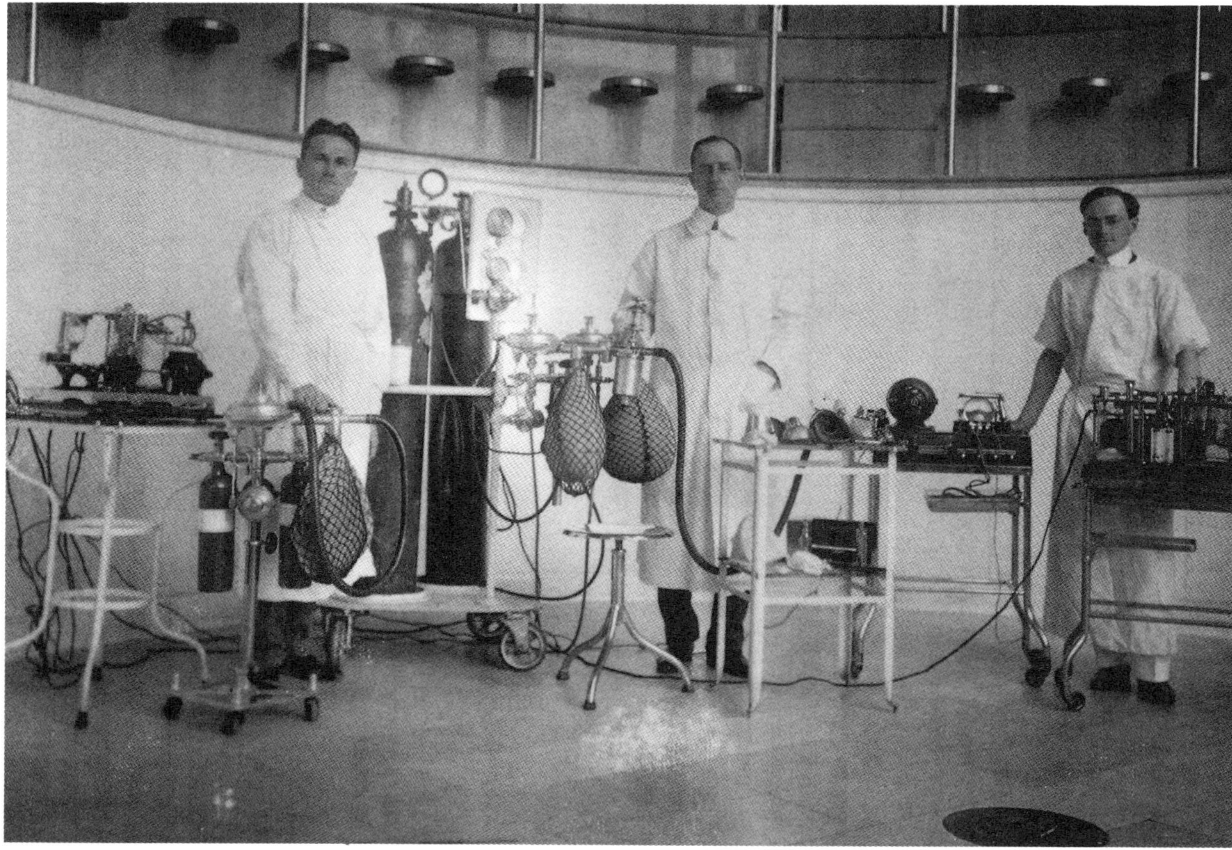

Figure 5. Operating room scene (left to right) W. Bourne, F.W. Nagle, G.M. Geldert (Ottawa), ca. 1915.

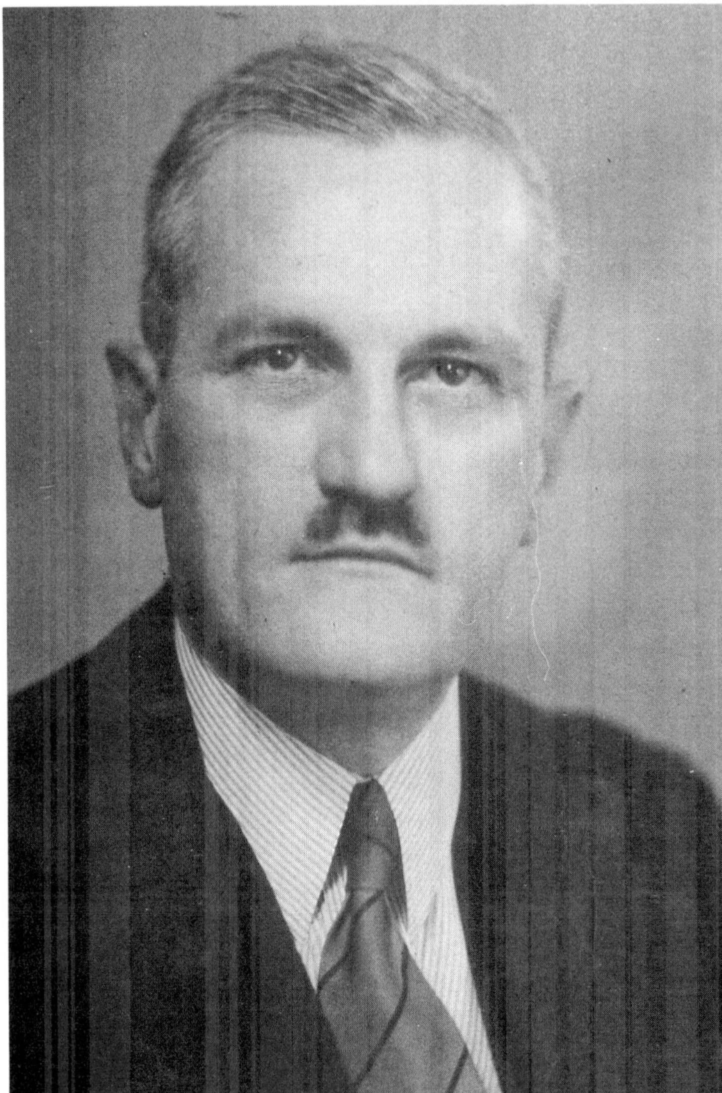

Figure 6. Portrait of Wesley Bourne during his middle years.

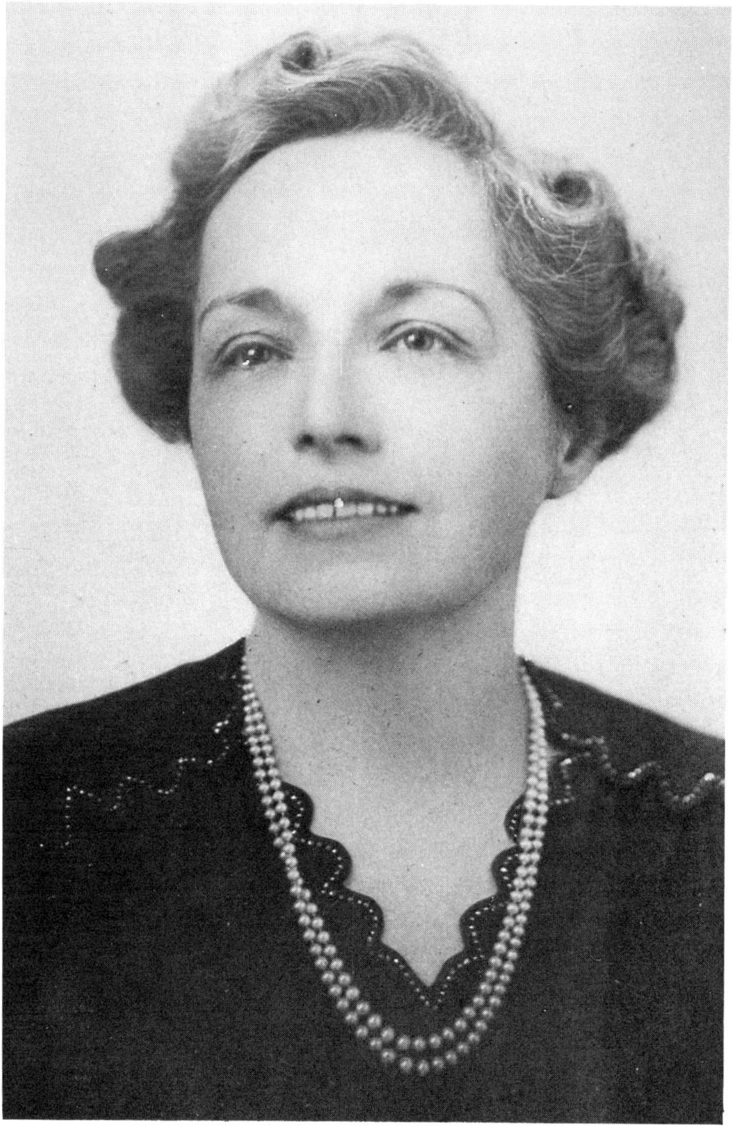

Figure 7. Portrait of Sara Bourne (née McGillis) during her middle years.

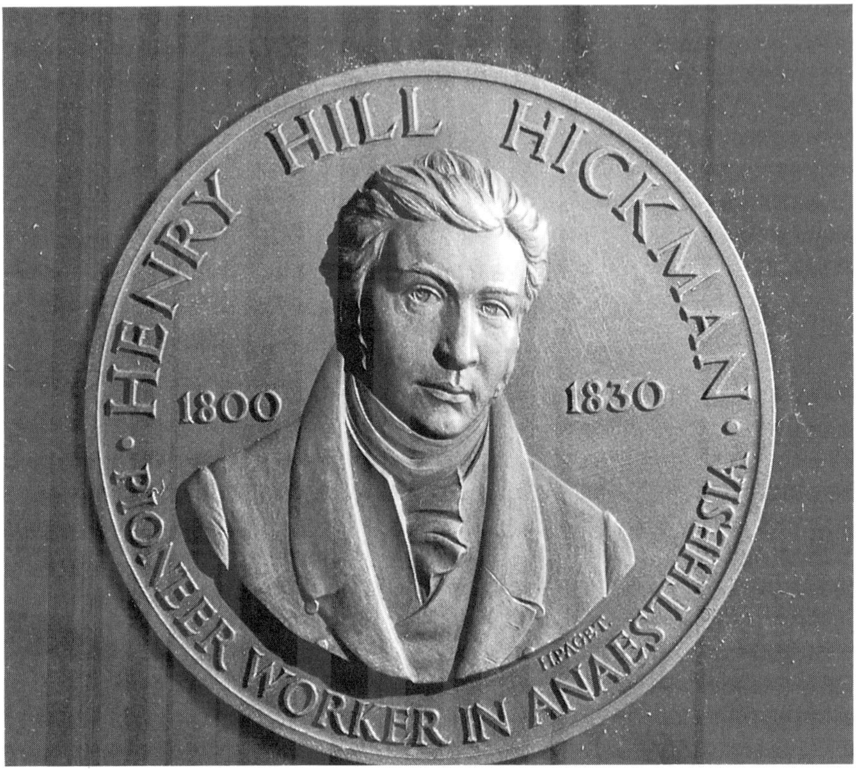

Figure 8. First Henry Hill Hickman Medal awarded to Wesley Bourne in 1935.

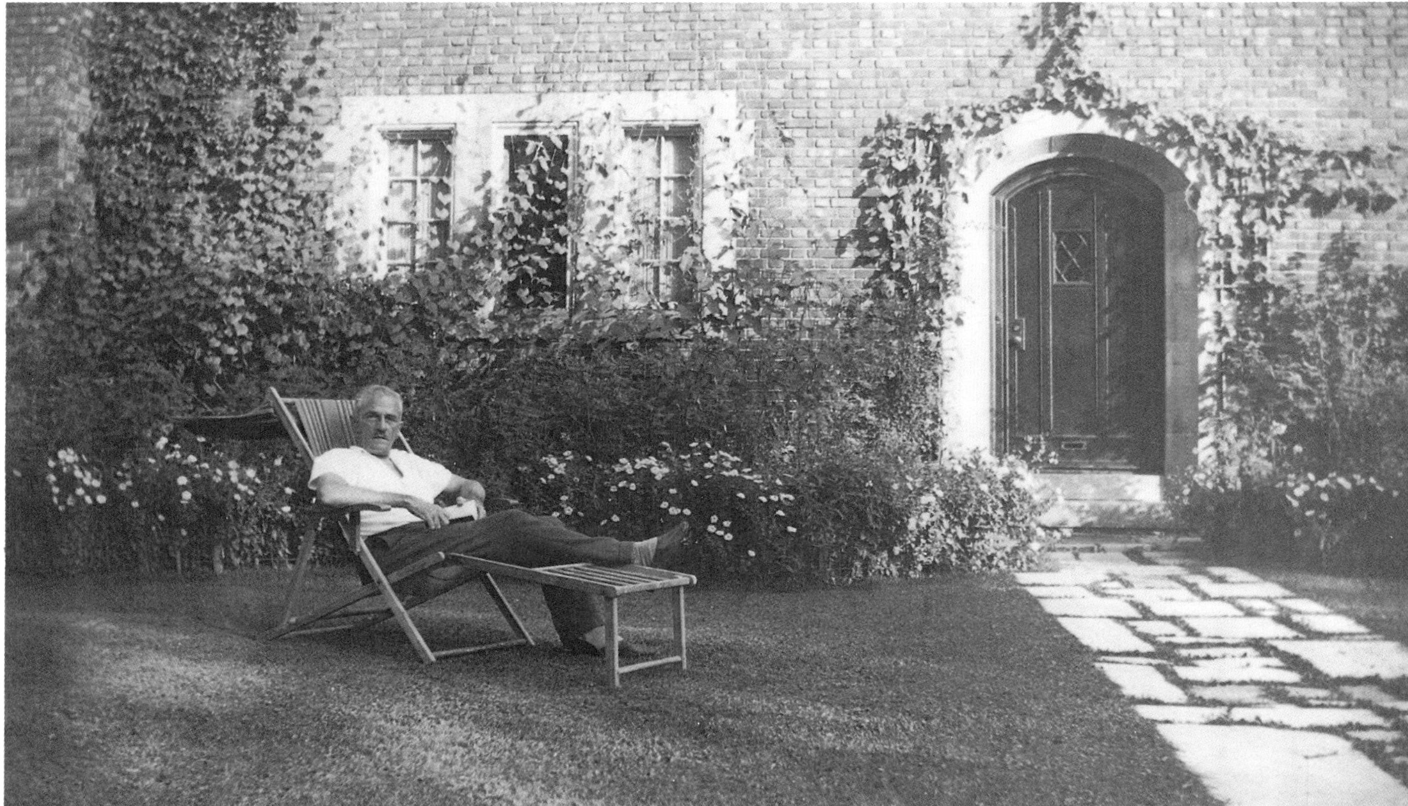

Figure 9. Wesley Bourne in his beloved garden, 32 Holton Avenue, 1937-39.

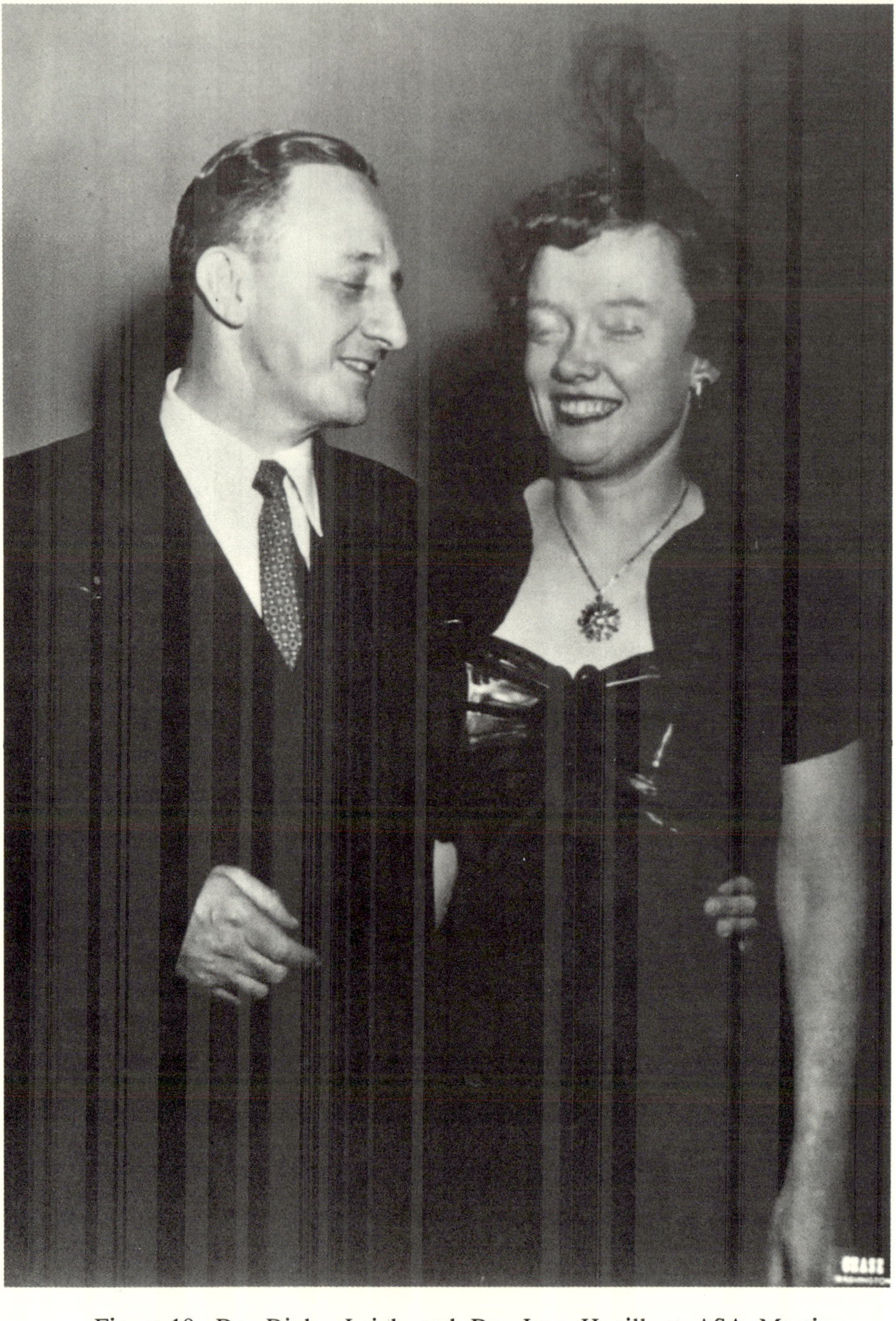

Figure 10. Dr. Digby Leigh and Dr. Jean Hugill at ASA Meeting; Washington, D.C., 1951.

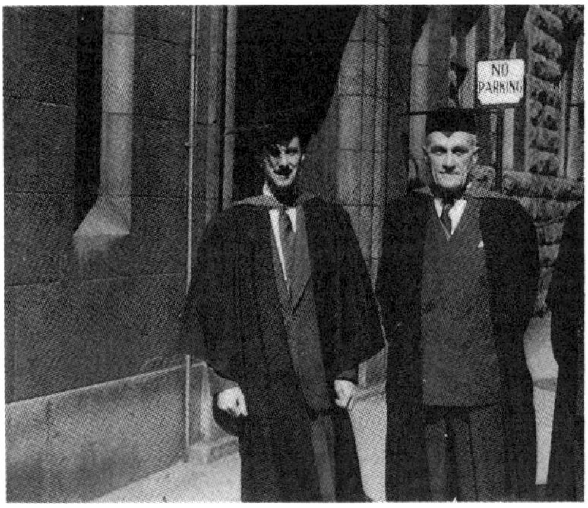

Figure 11a. Frank McCaffrey and Wesley Bourne, Graduating ceremony McGill campus (the first postgraduate diploma course, 1948).

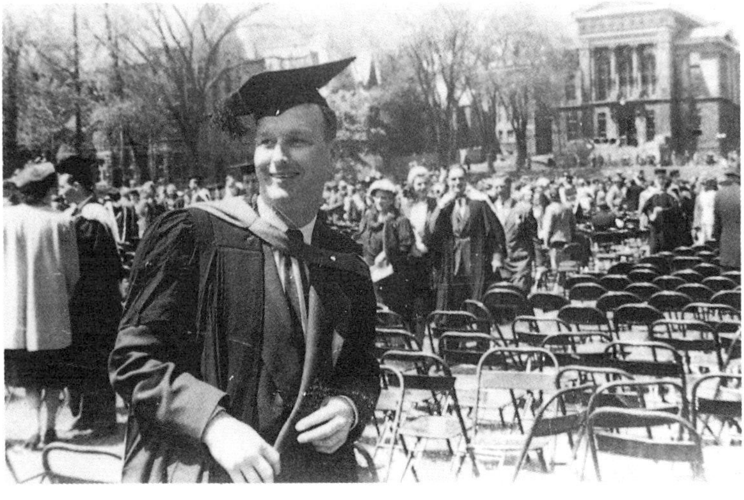

Figure 11b. Harold Kester, first postgraduate diploma course, 1948.

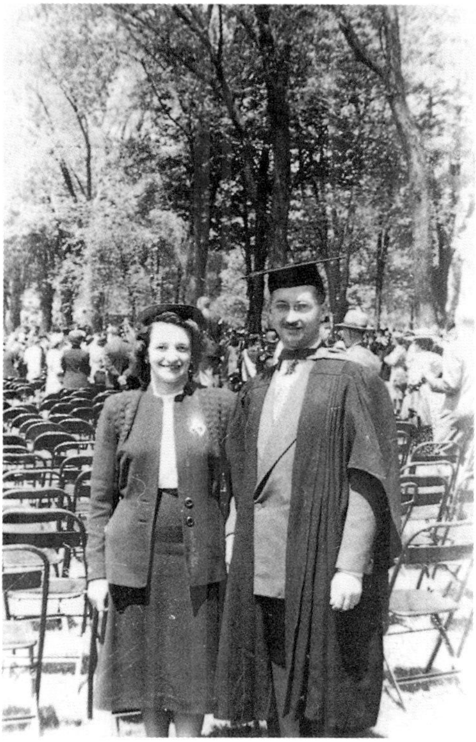

Figure 12. Harold Slater and his wife at graduation ceremony, McGill campus, first diploma course, 1948.

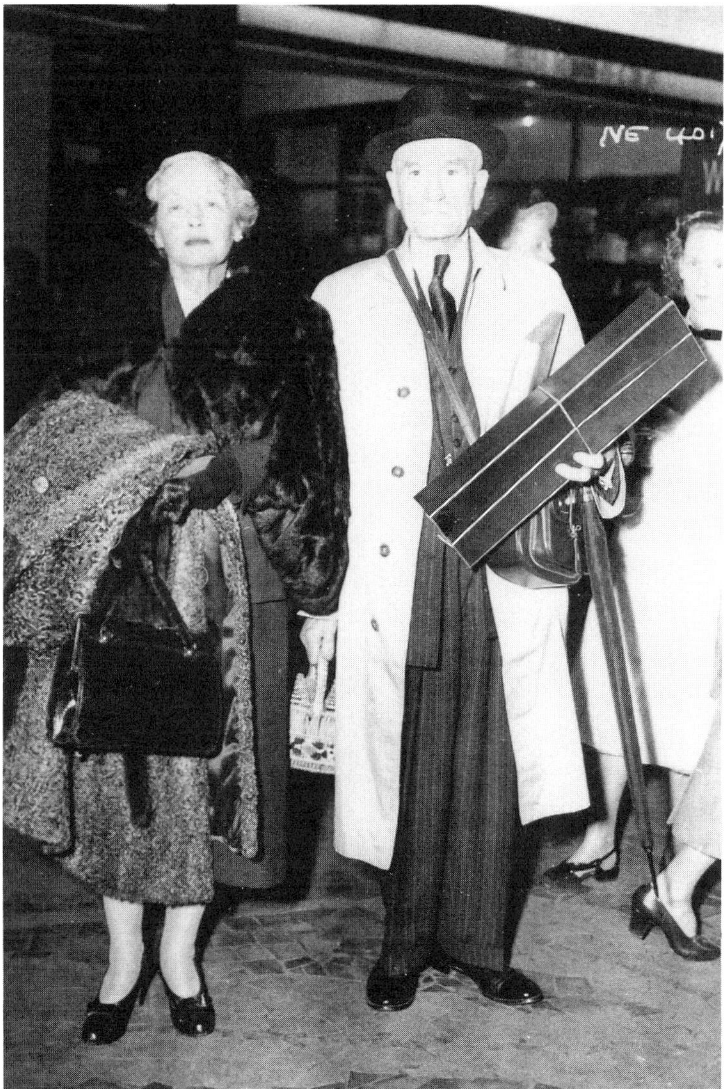

Figure 13. Wesley and Sara Bourne leaving for Paris in 1952.

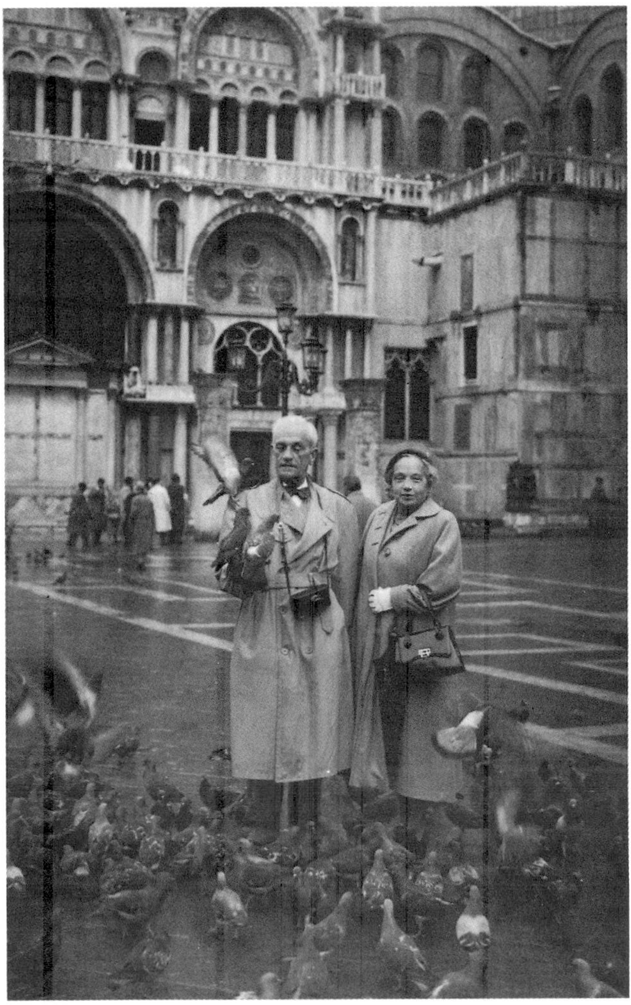

Figure 14. Wesley and Sara Bourne in Venice in 1954.

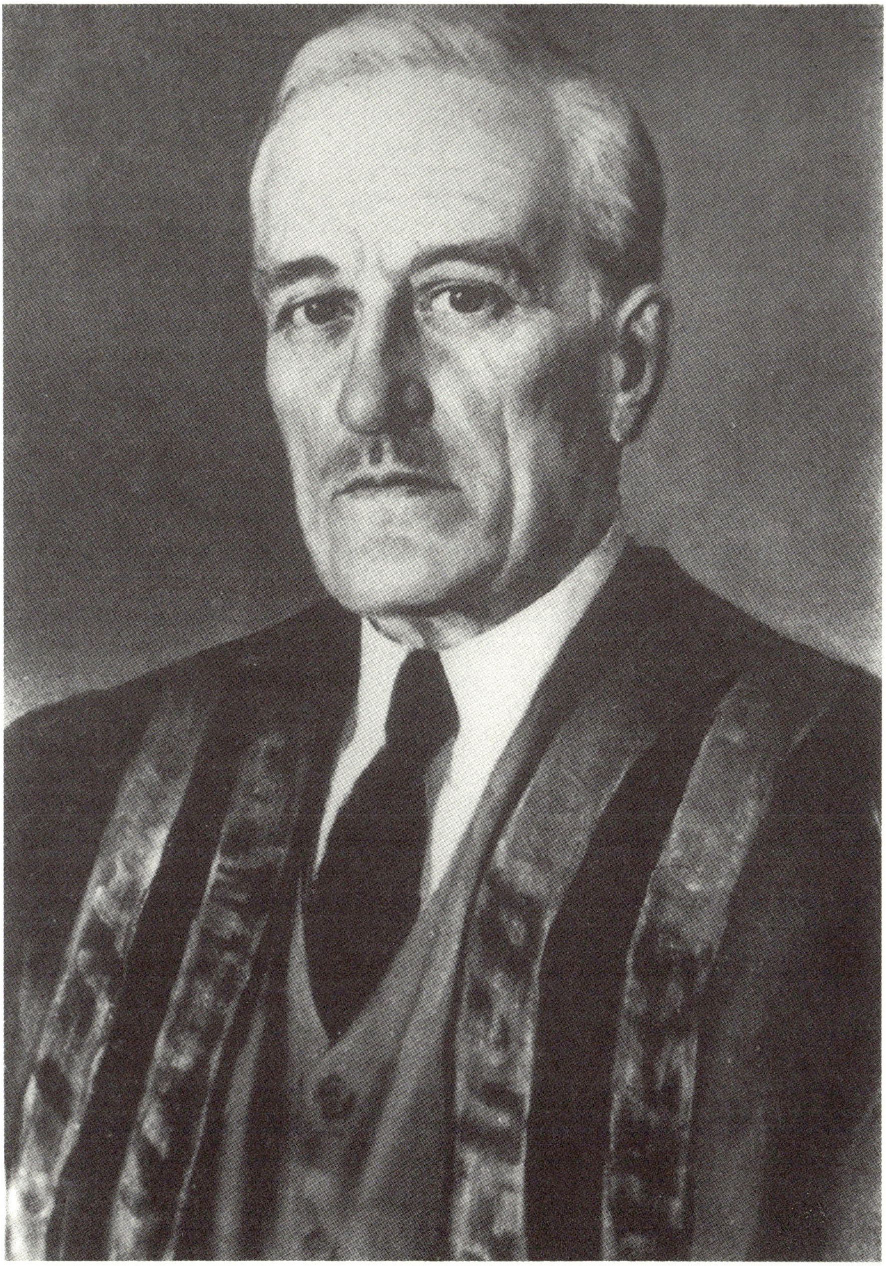

Figure 15. Portrait of Wesley Bourne by A. Sherriff Scott, presented to him by Québec anaesthetists in 1950. Portrait now in the McGill Department of Anesthesia.

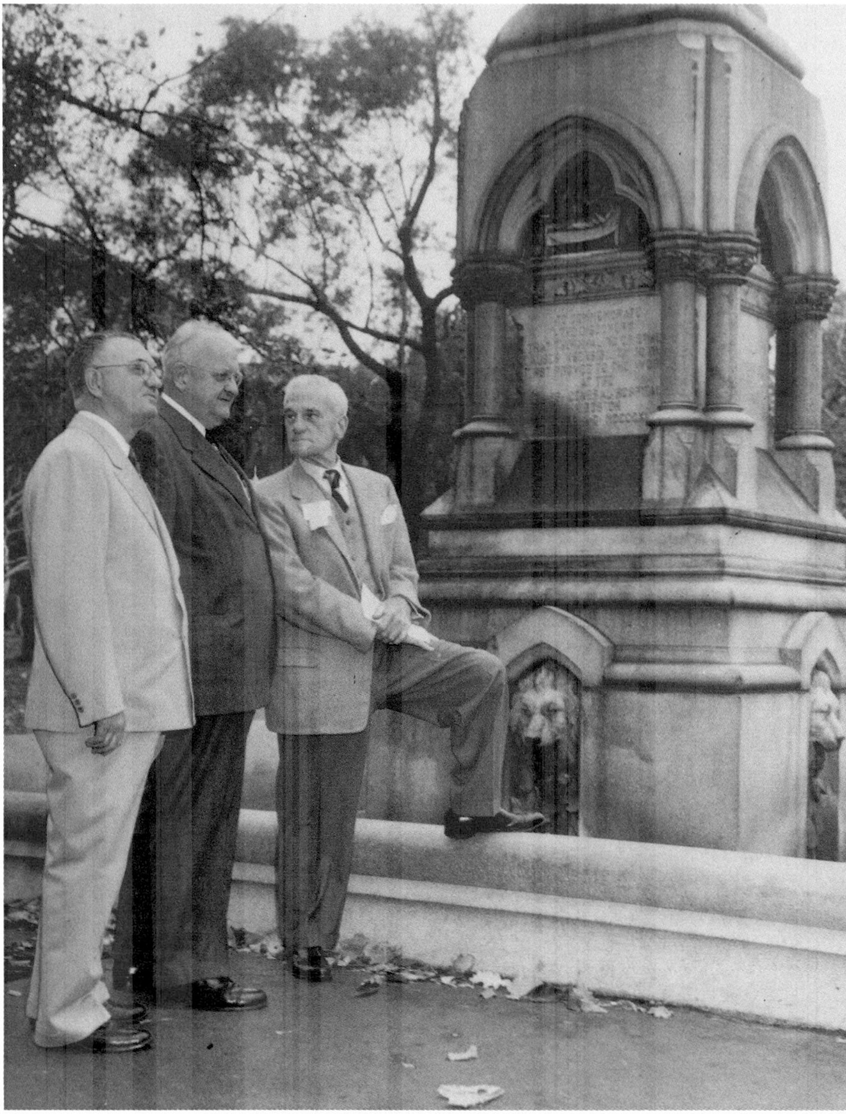

Figure 16. Wesley Bourne with John Lundy and Paul Wood at the Ether Memorial in Boston, Mass. on the occasion of the centennary celebration of Morton's introductory use of ether in anaesthesia. (Photo: Courtesy of Wood Library Museum)

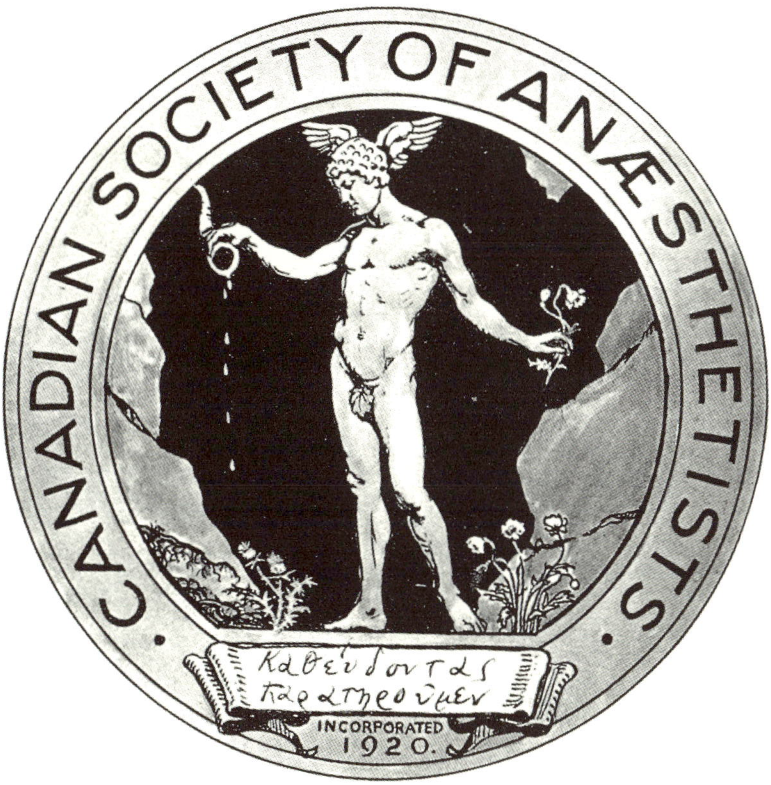

Figure 17. The Canadian Society of Anaesthetists' emblem depicting the God Hypnos, symbol of anæsthesia, in the Cave of Sleep. The motto translates as "we watch closely those who sleep." Drawn by Canadian artist A. Sheriff Scott.

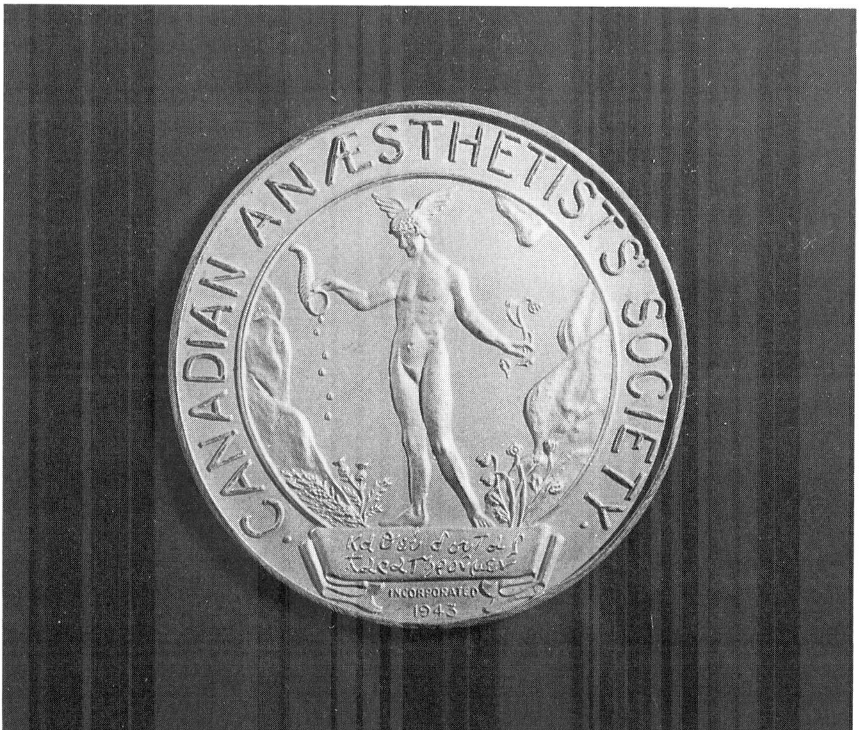

Figure 18. First gold medal of the Canadian Anæsthetists' Society for meritorious service awarded to Wesley Bourne in 1962. Depicts Society emblem with Hypnos.

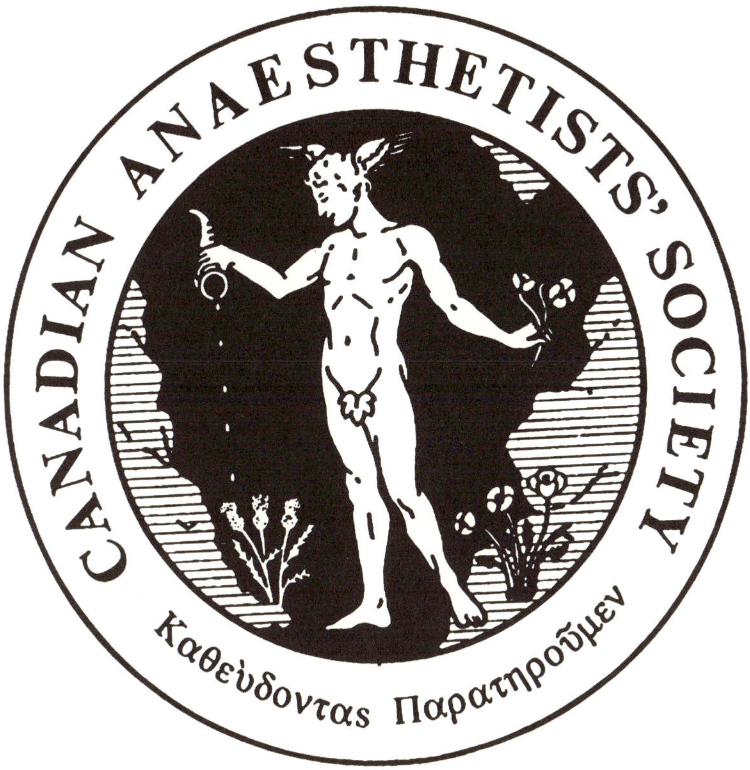

Figure 19. The logo of the Canadian Anæsthetists' Society, a stylized adaptation of the original 1920 emblem (Figure 17.)

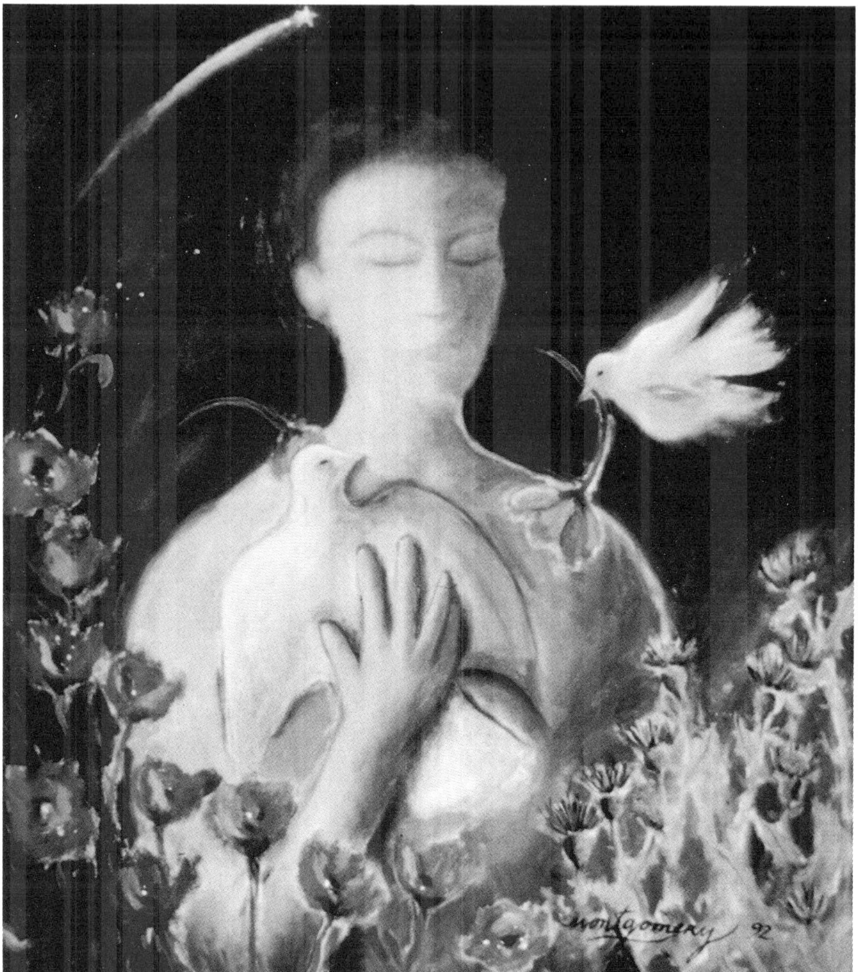

Figure 20. "Hypnos". Painting by Linda Montgomery unveiled at the 50th anniversary of the Canadian Anæsthetists' Society, 8 June, 1992.

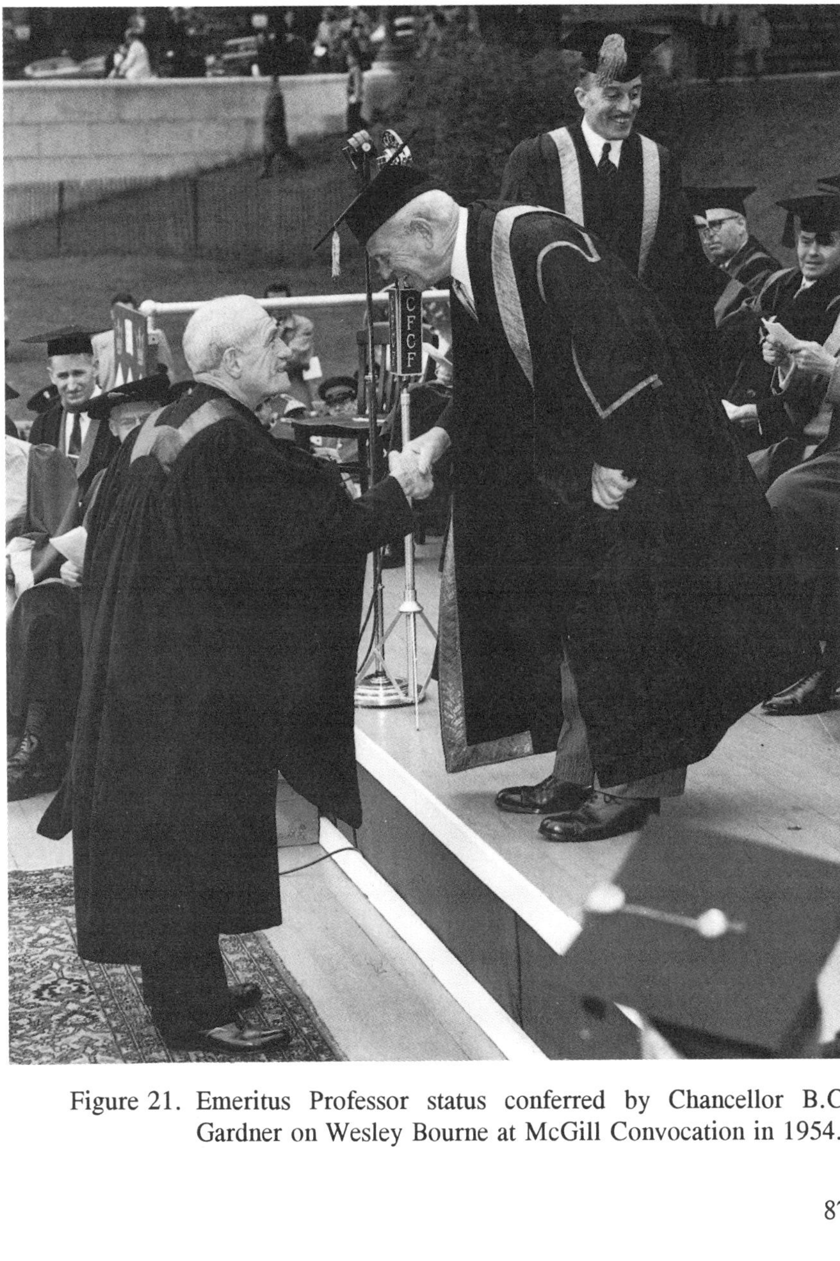

Figure 21. Emeritus Professor status conferred by Chancellor B.C. Gardner on Wesley Bourne at McGill Convocation in 1954.

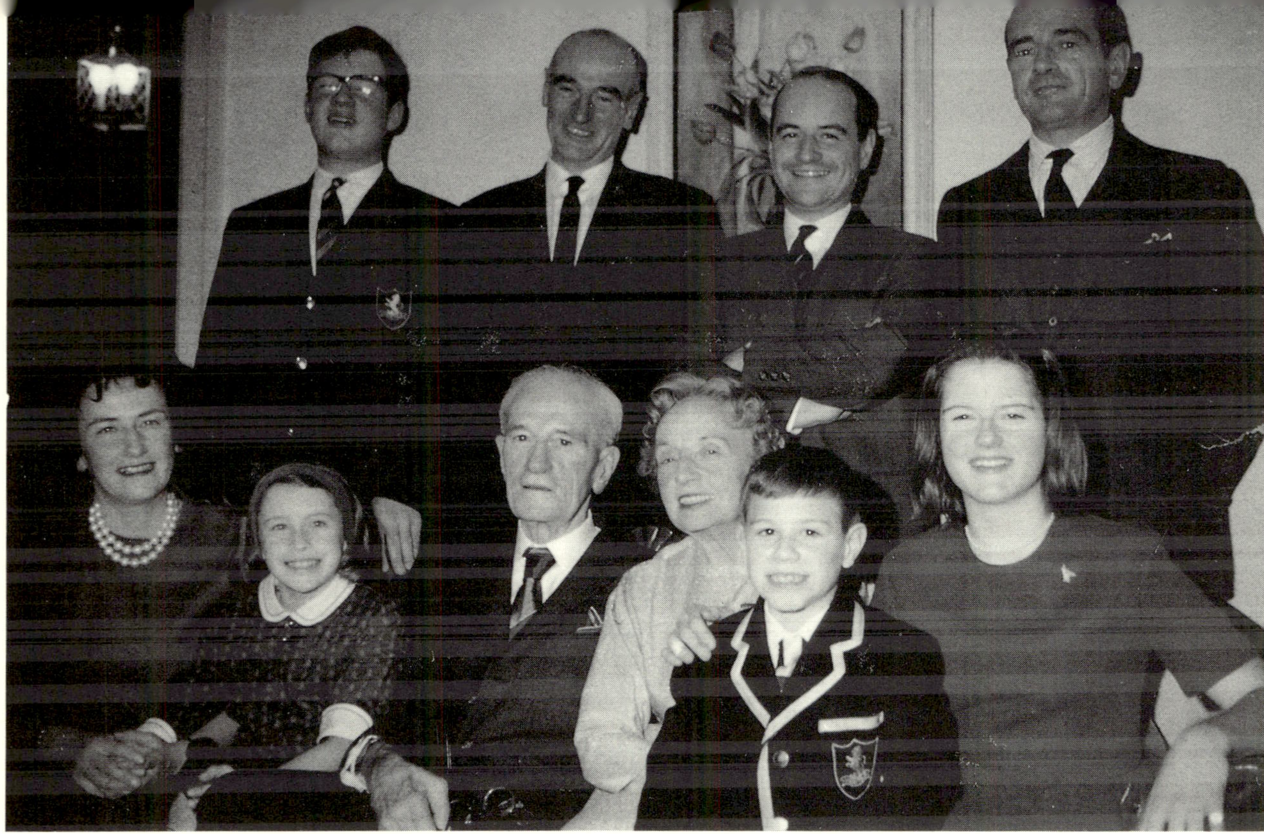

Figure 22. Bourne Family. Bottom left to right: Barbara Bourne (Krupski), Anne K. Bourne, Dr. Wesley Bourne, Mrs. Sara Bourne, Gerry Bourne, Sara Elspeth Bourne. Top left to right Thomas Sidney Wesley Bourne, James Douglas Bourne, Bobby Bourne, John Gilbert Bourne.

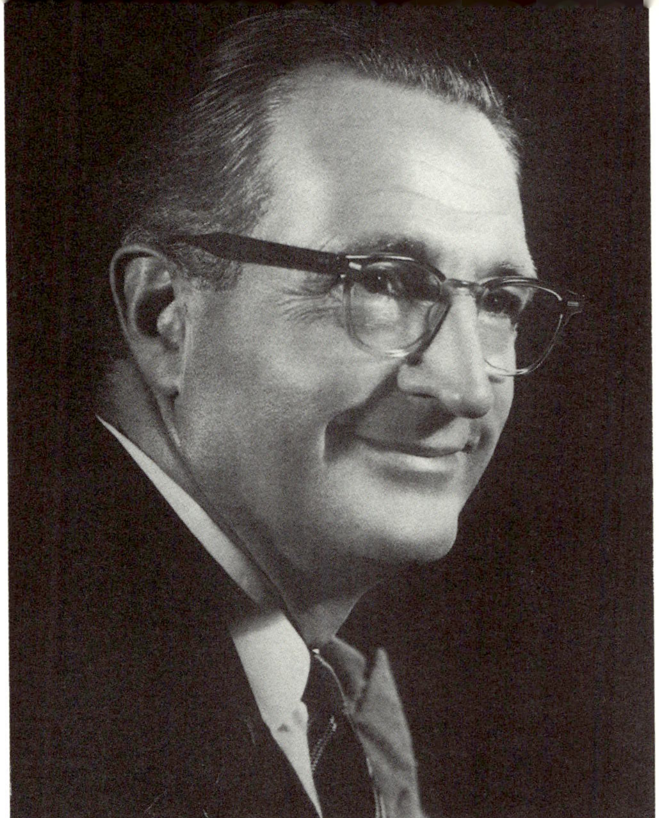

Figure 23. Dr. Richard G.B. Gilbert, Chair of the McGill Department of Anesthesia, 1957-70.

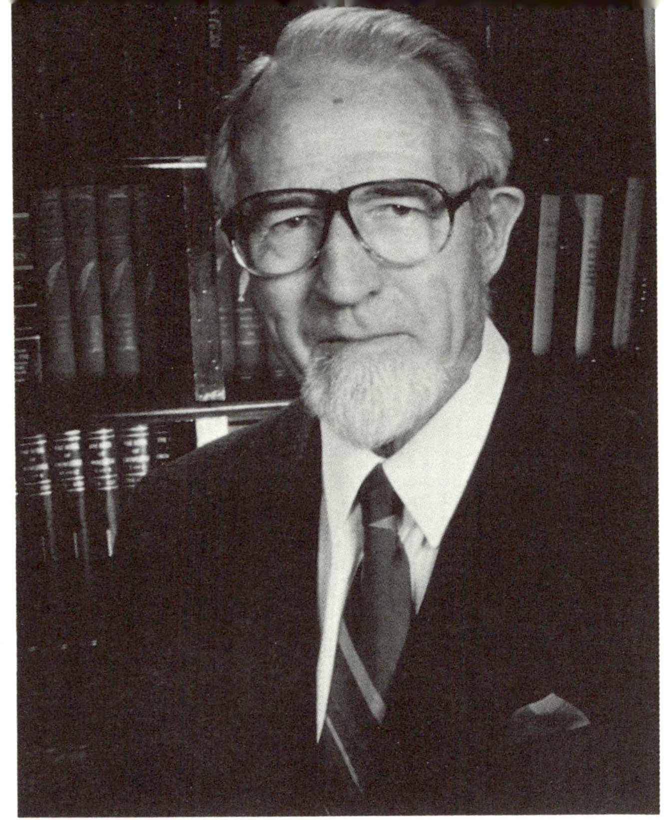

Figure 24. Dr. Phillip R. Bromage, Chair of the McGill Department of Anesthesia, 1970-76.

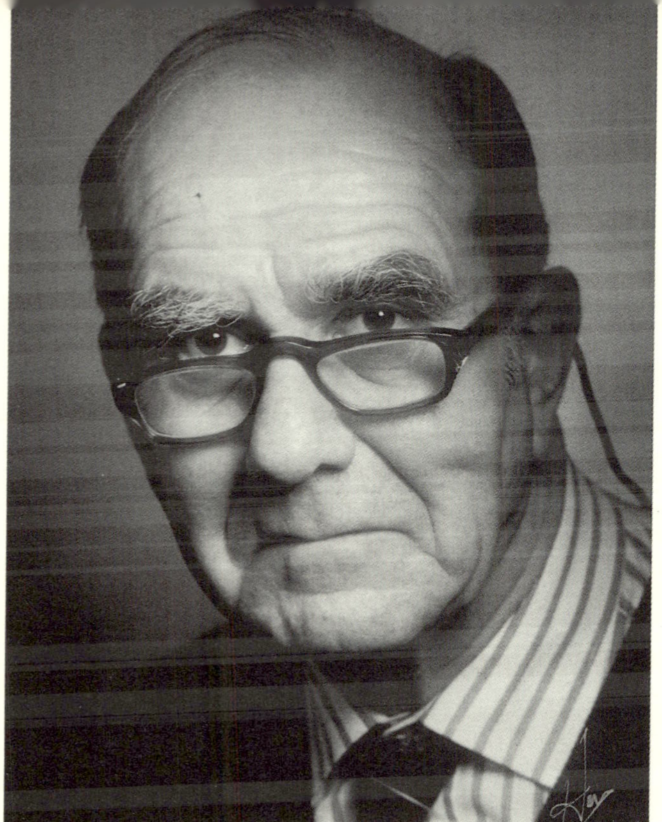

Figure 25. Dr. John W. Sandison, Chair of the McGill Department of Anesthesia, 1977-85.

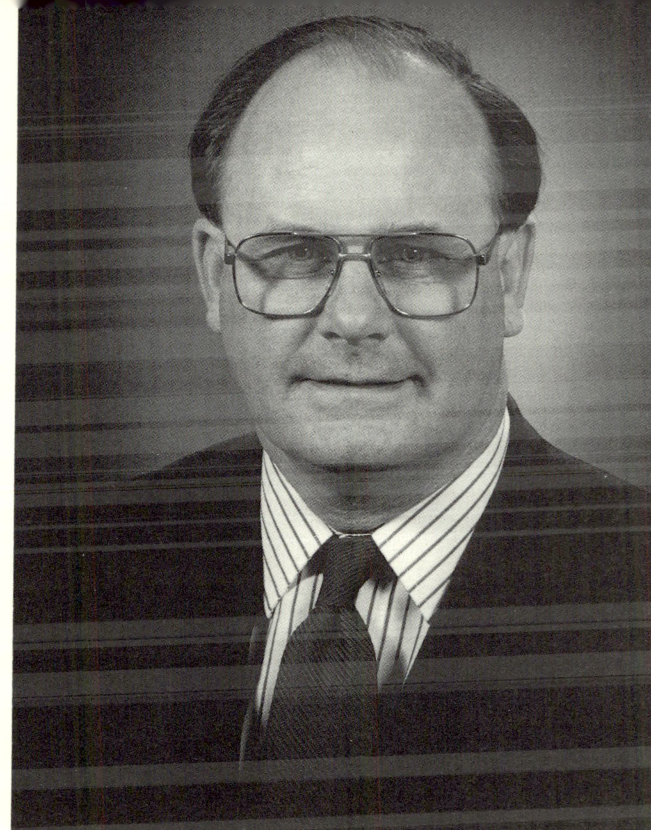

Figure 26. Dr. David R. Bevan, Chair of the McGill Department of Anesthesia, 1985-91.

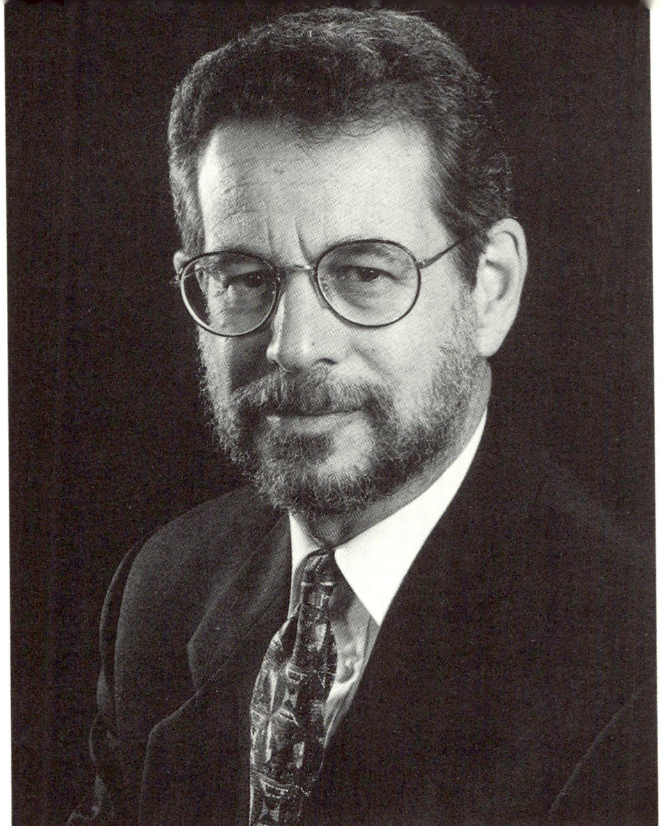

Figure 27. Dr. Gordon S. Fox, Acting Chair of the McGill Department of Anesthesia, 1992-94.

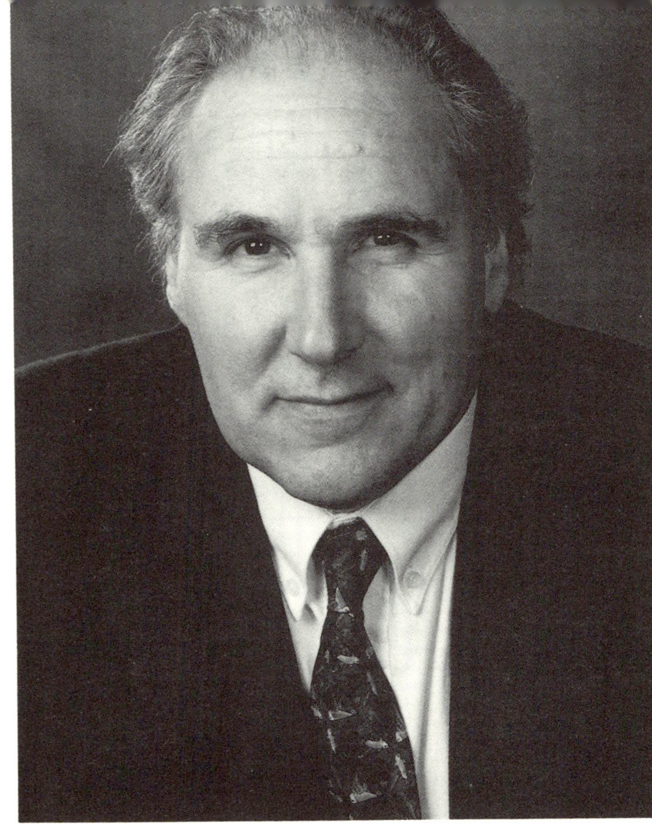

Figure 28. Dr. Francisco Carli, Chair of the McGill Department of Anesthesia, 1994- .

VI

Retirement Years (1950-65)

During Wesley Bourne's association with Montreal and McGill, the city and University had redefined their roles and relationships. European colonialism was ending and Quebec was embracing a new and different reality which would percolate through society for the next twenty or thirty years; vividly portrayed in Hugh McLennan's 1949 book, *Two Solitudes*. McGill had been transformed from a small, solidly Protestant school into a rapidly-growing, cosmopolitan institution. Public funding was needed to allow McGill to expand. The new political climate meant that the University had to refuse federal funding, but in the late 1950s provincial funding was forthcoming. The college-age population in Canada increased to one million by 1960 and two new French universities opened in Quebec. In the decade after his retirement, student enrolment reached almost ten times the number that it had been when Wesley Bourne entered McGill.

In the 1950s the Quiet Revolution, the search for social and cultural identity for French Quebec, was marked by the death of Premier Duplessis in 1959. The end of hte Duplessis era would fuel student unrest and foment change, culminating in the October Crisis of 1970. During this time, the French studies programme at McGill was emphasized, although the institution remained predominantly English in character. There had to be a major review of the curriculum when Collèges d'Enseignement Général et Professionnel (CEGEP) replaced the traditional college system in 1966, adding a year of education. English students began to leave the province to attend universities elsewhere to avoid this delay. Throughout McGill, traditions of research and teaching were pursued, even though evidence of change came in many areas. Federal support for student fellowship awards and Canada scholarships, initiated in 1956, lasted until 1994. The Redpath Library moved into a new building in 1953, the University Bookstore opened in its first home on McTavish in 1950 and the McGill University Press was established in the following year. Cyclotron research began to show results in the 1950s and computers were introduced on campus in 1959. The next year, McGill attracted almost a quarter of the available funds for medical research from the newly formed Medical Research Council of Canada. In 1962, Cyril James resigned, ending his twenty-two years as Principal. His successor, Harold Rocke Robertson was a surgeon and an astute businessman, who concerned himself mainly with rationalizing the administrative affairs of the University.

The McGill Department of Anesthesia was an integral part of the changes taking place throughout the University. On 1st June, 1950, immediately following Wesley Bourne's retirement, the chairmanship passed naturally to Dr. Harold R. Griffith; a charismatic leader with an aptitude for administration, but not a natural scientist. He had always seen the wisdom of Bourne's emphasis on research, and planned to keep the department on the same path. His own talents lay in international organization and the ability to attract funding to his department, so he recruited others to develop the research department and realize Wesley Bourne's ambitions. Edgar A. Pask, for one year, then Gordon Robson as the Wellcome Professor for the next ten years, came from England to enshrine basic scientific research in this department's mandate. To complement the strong clinical service component, clinical research was also encouraged, with the appointment in 1956 of Philip Bromage, also from England, a leading authority on epidural analgesia in childbirth. Links with pharmaceutical manufacturers were firm and when the new inhalational agent Fluothane, was introduced into Canada in 1956, the first clinical trials of the agent in North America were carried out by Gordon Robson in the McGill department.

Dr. Dick Gilbert took over the departmental chair from Harold Griffith. He had been involved in the Ciba meetings and expanded the teaching mandate. He introduced the Annual Refresher Course, which was announced in the *American Society of Anesthesiologists Newsletter* as the "McGill University postgraduate course in anesthesiology." The first course took place from September 14 to 26, 1959. It was held immediately before the certification and fellowship examinations as a review for part-time anæsthetists and consisted of one week of lectures followed by an optional week of clinical teaching. In 1960, the Review Course was again held, from September 11 to 16, with the mornings devoted to study or clinical observation and the afternoons spent in lectures. The course was open to general practitioner anæsthetists as well as examination candidates, at a fee of only $35. In the next year, the refresher course was moved forward to the last week in May, a place in the University calendar that it has since retained. The clinical teaching was soon removed from this forum, allowing the interactive lecture format of the modern annual refresher course to develop.

Although Wesley Bourne retired from the University faculty, he continued to give anæsthetics in the Montreal hospitals for a little longer. Then, the World Health Organization offered him the opportunity to go to Paris for fifteen months. Widespread recognition of his postgraduate training programme had resulted in the French government asking him to assist them by organizing a similar specialist training at the University of Paris. He worked with Professor

P. Moulonguet, a surgeon, who had visited Montreal two years previously. Characteristically, Wesley Bourne prepared for his trip by studying French culture under Professor André Rigault of the Department of Romance Languages at McGill and formerly of the Sorbonne, Paris. On 14th October, 1952 Mrs. Bourne accompanied him to New York, where they boarded the French liner "Liberté" to sail to France[1]. While he was in Europe, Harold Griffith was organizing the World Federation of Societies of Anæsthesiologists (WFSA) and he invited Wesley Bourne to be a member of the international organizing committee which met in Belgium in 1953.

This Federation grew out of the Anesthetists' Travel Club, of which Harold Griffith was one of the founding members. However, the group was disbanded in 1952 and then revived as the Academy of Anesthesiology in 1954, with Wesley Bourne and Harold Griffith amongst its charter members. Membership continues to be limited and is by invitation only. Its purpose was to foster and encourage the advancement of education and research in the arts and sciences of anæsthesia. These were goals which were important to both men, and Harold Griffith was able to obtain financial backing from the International Anesthesia Research Society to make the development of the WFSA viable. He fully understood that funding was pivotal to the success of any organization, whereas Wesley Bourne was probably less interested in such matters. The two Canadians met in Brussels, where the committee debated what sort of organization would be acceptable to all the diverse national specialist societies. They had sent out a questionnaire to the existing societies to find out how many anæsthetists practised in different countries and the status of these anæsthetists. They received replies from 7,000 society members in twenty-three countries; including 4,000 in the United States, 888 in the United Kingdom and 490 in Canada. This was a healthy start to the formation of this international venture which is now responsible for the World Congress of Anæsthesiologists (WCA), that is held in a different country every four years. The second meeting took place in Toronto, and Montreal is the venue chosen for the WCA in the year 2,000.

On his return to Montreal, further honours awaited Wesley Bourne.

---

[1] The French liner "Liberté" was reported in the Montreal newspapers, but conflicts with J.D. Bourne's recollection that his parents sailed in "RMS Queen Elizabeth." There is a photograph which confirms the latter and it is possible that Dr. and Mrs. Bourne returned home on the "Liberté" as they had talked about that ship.

Chancellor B.C. Gardner conferred an emeritus professorship on him on 29th May, 1954, marked by placing a scarlet cloth hood around his shoulders during a two-and-a-half-hour convocation ceremony. The correspondence relating to this appointment was retained in the hospital records.

April 29, 1954

Dear Dr Bourne,

I am pleased to inform you that the Board of Governors at its last meeting appointed you Emeritus Professor of Anæsthesia in appreciation of your long and distinguished service to the Faculty of Medicine and the University.

Yours sincerely,

Bursar and Secretary of the Board of Governors.

May 1, 1954

Dear Mr Bentley,

I am pleased to acknowledge the receipt of your letter of April 29, 1954 informing me that the Board of Governors of McGill university, at its last meeting, appointed me Emeritus Professor of Anæsthesia.

Will you please convey to the Board my deep appreciation.

Yours faithfully,

Wesley Bourne.

Accordingly, the last record was entered on Wesley Bourne's staff record: Emeritus Professor of Anæsthesia, 14th April, 1954.

In 1954, Wesley Bourne saw the flourishing Canadian Anæsthetists' Society begin publication of its own journal, *The Canadian Anæsthetists' Society Journal*. Dr. Roderick A. Gordon was its first editor with an editorial board of Drs. Alan B. Noble, Louis Lamoureux and E.A. Gain. This journal was published quarterly and replaced the *News Letter* (which had served for several years to inform members across Canada about society activities) and the *Proceedings/Compte-rendus* (which contained papers read at meetings in the previous two years) of the society. By 1962 the journal was well established, with Dr. Gordon continuing as editor, an editorial board of four members, and a regional board of eleven members representing anæsthetists in cities across Canada. This was the first year in which the title appeared in English and

French as *The Canadian Anæsthetists' Society Journal/Journal de la Société Canadienne des Anesthétistes*.

Five years after official retirement, Wesley Bourne was still in demand as a speaker. He was a guest lecturer at the Medical Society of the State of North Carolina annual meeting, the Trent Historical Society of Duke University and the Maryland Society of Anesthesiologists. His topics were philosophical, entitled "Anæsthesia evolving," "Humanity and science in anæsthesia" and "The spirit in anæsthesia." He appeared in the programme of the Canadian Anæsthetists' Society annual meeting, held in Toronto in June 1955, as chairman of a round table discussion on hypotension in anæsthesia and as an after-dinner speaker. This was the year in which the book, *Mysterious Waters to Guard*, was published, bringing together Wesley Bourne's most important publications and speeches in one volume.

The American Society of Anesthesiologists elected Wesley Bourne to honorary membership in 1957. In the announcement in their *Newsletter*, a very touching tribute was expressed: "No man has contributed more to the development of the specialty in Canada and the United States. He is known and beloved by all the members of the ASA. Certainly, no one is more deserving of this honor than Dr. Bourne." One of the finest hours was yet to come in 1962: when Wesley Bourne, at the age of 76 years, was awarded the first Canadian Anæsthetists' Society Gold Medal for meritorious service in anæsthesia. He stood with his two friends, Drs. Harry Shields of Toronto and Harold Griffith of Montreal for this honour. Dr. Rod Gordon's words on this occasion bear repeating: "While the award in each case is made for outstanding service in their professional careers it is undoubtedly true that the same selection could have been made on the basis of the personal love and esteem which these three men command in the hearts of the anæsthetists of Canada." (*Can Anæsth Soc J* 1962;9:371-4). These two tributes from North American anæsthetists summarize the whole of this man's story.

For most of his life, Wesley Bourne seemed to have an iron constitution which served him well, but he began to suffer from Parkinson's disease. The inevitable downhill nature of this affliction was hard to take and very frustrating for him, but, in the main, he was remarkably cheerful throughout his ordeal, which lasted more than five years. There was always a religious streak in him. He was sentimental when listening to the hymns of his boyhood on the Sunday evening services on the radio and, as a student, taught Sunday school at St.

John's Anglican Church in Montreal. His conversion to Roman Catholicsm came about as a result of the influence of "Uncle Jimmy," and was before the time that he met Sara, his wife. However, he was an agnostic during his working career. Towards the end of his life, he returned to the Roman Catholic Church. Using sound judgment, Sara decided that, considering his whole life, she would abandon the usual Roman Catholic custom of entwining rosary beads in his hands. His death came on Friday, 26th February, 1965 in his 79th year, in the Grace Dart Hospital, one of the small hospitals in Montreal that he loved so well. A funeral service was held at the Church of the Ascension of Our Lord at 9.30 a.m. on Monday 1st March, 1965. Even he, like everyone, perhaps had a little vanity. He told his wife, Sara, that all he wanted on his tombstone was "Wesley Bourne MD" with the years spanning his life, and, that is the way that it is.

VII

PUBLICATIONS

Wesley Bourne was a bibliophile. He loved books and left a wealth of his own publications for those who would follow. These books span the years between the pioneering days of early Canadian anæsthesia and the specialization of the present. Without them, the history of the evolution of anæsthesia would lack much: having them provides a colourful tapestry of the changing milieu in which the McGill Department of Anesthesia has flourished.

In the thirty-five years extending from Wesley Bourne's initiation in the Department of Pharmacology, throughout his career in anæsthesia and into his retirement years, he authored 138 publications. Generally, he was the sole author, but his research collaborators co-authored investigative reports. Some of his close clinical associates were also occasional co-authors. Most are papers read at medical or specialist anæsthesia meetings, as was the custom of the day. In this way, written copies of the lecture would be circulated to reach a wider audience. Consequently, it was not unusual for the same paper to be reproduced in two different journals to expand the readership, so at least eleven of Wesley Bourne's addresses at major meetings appear concurrently, in identical form, in two journals in North America or in the United Kingdom. His most productive period was in the 1920s and 1930s when he was an active laboratory investigator and travelled widely to present reports of his work at major meetings in Canada (Ottawa, Montreal, Toronto, Winnipeg), the United States (Columbus Ohio, Chicago, Atlantic City, Washington DC, Boston) and the United Kingdom (Glasgow, Nottingham, London).

Early topics were related to physiology and pharmacology: temperature, body fluids, hepatic and renal dysfunction and acidosis of anæsthesia. Others were clinical: anæsthesia for obstetrics, emergency abdominal surgery, and gall bladder surgery. His style was a model for the contemporary writer to follow. In a concise and organized fashion, he laid out the research plan and results, or the clinical problem and its management. Abstracts were not generally used to introduce the article, rather, the concluding paragraph summarized the content. Sometime later, this paragraph was moved to the first page of an article, the position which has now become familiar. The introduction of a French language abstract in the Canadian journals also took place in the 1940s. As Wesley Bourne's career matured, his role moved more to teaching and administration, so the emphasis in his publications shifted into the same areas. Overall, his publications provided the model for the successful performance of various aspects of anæsthesia, as an individual or within an organizational setting: research, clinical care, teaching and administration. Although his papers were abstracted in French journals and he included many illustrative quotations in Greek, Latin and other languages, it is still surprising to see a few articles entirely in German, French and Spanish. In later years, his philosophical interjections became more prominent and could be understood by the lay person and the classical scholar, as well as the specialist in anæsthesia.

The journals to which he contributed tell their own story. Specialist anæsthetic journals were not available at the start of the 1920s, so his papers were published in the Proceedings of individual societies or the *Canadian Medical Association Journal.* Wesley Bourne disseminated his papers to all the available journals of the time, so that he appeared as a contributor to twelve journals in the 1920s and to thirty-eight journals eventually. He appealed to a varied audience which included nurses, students, obstetricians, pharmacologists, and physiologists, as well as anæsthetists. Two papers were awarded prizes in the "Best essay" competition in the *British Journal of Anæsthesia* in 1935 and the prize competition of the Société d'Anesthésie et Analgésie in 1936.

After his retirement, Wesley Bourne collected his addresses and essays in a book, *Mysterious Waters to Guard,* dedicated to his wife, Sara Beatrice McGillis. Perhaps the title reflects the unknown about anæsthesia or maybe it related to the physiological environment which he knew changed so much during anæsthesia. The book includes the fascinating sermon "Cultivate your Garden" which cannot be found easily elsewhere, and the memorial address, "Francis Hoeffer McMechan: An Apotheosis" which was enclosed with, but not indexed in the 1940 *Current Researches in Anesthesia and Analgesia.* Falconer Hill's review of the book for the *British Journal of Anæsthesia* was not especially complimentary because he failed to see the historical value of the text and instead related it to anæsthetic practice of his own day, distanced from the content of the book by as much as twenty or thirty years. Although the subject matter has, indeed, been superseded by changing clinical profiles, better understanding of anæsthetic-induced derangements, technological change and a pharmacopæia of new drugs, the principles of practice remain the same.

The special joy that comes from reading these manuscripts is three-fold: they forge links between modern practice and early Canadian anæsthesia, lay bare the foundations of the McGill Department of Anesthesia and are a stimulus to reading classical literature. Perhaps there is also a message: that we must understand the present status of anæsthesia and manipulate its future. Indeed, the 1956 article, "On the duties of the anesthesiologist as a physician," (*Curr Res Anesth Analg* 1956;35:115-22) has been used as a reference in two recent publications in *Anesthesia and Analgesia* (1991;73:221-45 and 1992;74:327).

The following bibliography is as complete as possible. However, the journals in the early part of this century paid scant regard to the completeness of their indices and computerized database retrieval belongs to a later period. It was certainly "Fun" trying to trace as many of these as possible, and to appreciate the changing format of editorial styles as they developed towards current expectations. Some publications may remain elusive:

1920s

1. Bourne W, Duncan JW. Nitrous oxide-oxygen analgesia and anæsthesia in obstetrics. *Can Med Assoc J* 1921;11:818-22. (Presentation: Montreal Medico-Chirurgical Society, April, 1921 and Hamilton Medical Society, 6th April, 1921).

2. Stehle RL, Bourne W. The anesthetic properties of pure ether. *JAMA* 1922;79:375-6. (Presentation: Canadian Medical Association and Canadian Society of Anæsthetists Joint Meeting, Winnipeg, 20th June, 1922).

3. Stehle RL, Bourne W, Barbour HG. Effects of ether anesthesia alone or preceded by morphine upon the alkali metabolism of the dog. *J Biol Chem* 1922;53:341-8. (Presentation: Canadian Society of Anæsthetists Meeting Winnipeg June, 1922).

4. Bourne W. Retrospect: Nitrous oxide. *Can Med Assoc J* 1923:13:50.

5. Bourne W. Retrospect: Hypertonic solutions. *Can Med Assoc J* 1923; 13:188-9. (Presentation: Osler Reporting Society, 20th December, 1922).

6. Bourne W, Stehle RL. Methylene chloride in anæsthesia. *Can Med Assoc J* 1923;13:432-3. (Presentation: Canadian Society of Anæsthetists Meeting, Montreal, June, 1923).

7. Bourne W. On the teaching of anæsthesia to medical students. *Br J Anæsth*

1923;1:74-8. (Presentation: Canadian Society of Anæsthetists Meeting, Winnipeg, June, 1922).

8. Bourne W. On the teaching of anesthesia to medical students. *Curr Res Anesth Analg* 1923;2:197-9. (Presentation: National Anesthesia Research Society Congress of Anesthetists Joint Meeting with Interstate and New York Anesthetists, Columbus, Ohio, 30th October - 1st November, 1922). (Also published in the *British Journal of Anæsthesia* 1923;1:74-8)

9. Barbour HG, Bourne W. Heat regulation and water exchange. IV. The influence of ether in dogs. *Am J Physiol* 1924;67:399-410. (Presentation: Canadian Society of Anæsthetists, Montreal, 12th June, 1923). (Thesis for MSc. McGill University, Montreal)

10. Bourne W, Stehle RL The excretion of phosphoric acid during anesthesia. *JAMA* 1924;83:117-8. (Presentation: Congress of Anesthetists, Chicago, 1924).

11. Stehle RL Bourne W. Concerning the mechanism of acidosis in anesthesia. *J Biol Chem* 1924;60:17-29. (Presentation: Mid-Western Society of Anesthetists' Meeting, Columbus, Ohio, 1923).

12. Barbour HG, Bourne W. Concerning the effects of anesthetics on body temperature and blood solids at various environmental conditions. *Curr Res Anesth Analg* 1924;3:116-20.

13. Barbour HG, Bourne W. Concerning the effects of anesthetics on body temperature and blood solids at various environmental conditions (continued). *Curr Res Anesth Analg* 1924;3:145-9. (Presentation: 3rd Annual Meeting, Canadian Society of Anæsthetists, Montreal, 12th-14th June 1923 and Presentation: 2nd Annual Congress, National Anesthesia Research Society Joint Meeting with the Interstate, Mid-Western and Chicago Anesthetists, Chicago, 22nd-24th October, 1923).

14. Bourne W. Anæsthesia in obstetrics. *Can Med Assoc J* 1924;14:702-3. (Presentation: Montreal Medico-Chirurgical Society, Montreal, 2nd May, 1924).

15. Bourne W. Anæsthesia in acute abdominal operations. *Can Med Assoc J*

1924;14:835-6. (Presentation: Canadian Medical Association, Ottawa, June, 1924).

16. Bourne W. The relation between the width of the pupil and the carbon dioxide content of the blood. *Can Med Assoc J* 1924;14:411-2. (Presentation: Osler Reporting Society, 22nd February, 1924).

17. Bourne W. Abstract: Anæsthesia in obstetrics (*Can Med Assoc J* 1924; 14:702-3). *Br J Anæsth* 1924;2:89.

18. Bourne W. Blood concentration and body temperature in anæsthesia. *Br J Anæsth* 1924;2:36-9. (Presentation: Canadian Society of Anæsthetists, Ottawa, 17th June, 1924).

19. Stehle RL, Bourne W, Lozinsky E. Uber die pharmakologische wirkung von athylenoxyd. *Archiv fur Experimentelle Pathologie und Pharmakologie* 1924;104:82-6.

20. Bourne W. Some recent advances in anesthesia: Presidential Address, Associated Anesthetists of the United States and Canada, 1925. *Curr Res Anesth Analg* 1925;4:259-66. (Presentation: 4th Annual Congress of Anesthetists, Associated Anesthetists of the United States and Canada, International Anesthesia Research Society Joint Meeting, Atlantic City, 25th-28th May. 1925).

21. Stehle RL Bourne W. The effect of pituitary extract on the secretion and composition of the urine. *J Physiol* 1925;60:229-36.

22. Bourne W. On the disposition of ether in the body. *Can Med Assoc J* 1925;15:84-5.

23. Bourne W. The hormone of oestrus. *Can Med Assoc J* 1925;15:171-3. (Presentation: Osler Reporting Society, 28th November, 1924).

24. Bourne W. The influence of diathermy in anæsthesia on body temperature, blood concentration, and acidosis. *Br J Anæsth.* 1926;4;87-91.

25. Bourne W. On an attempt to alleviate the acidosis of anæsthesia. *Proc Roy Soc Med* 1926;19 (Section of Anæsthetics): 49-51. (Presentation: Royal

Society of Medicine, London, England, 15th luly, 1926 and British Medical Association Meeting Nottingham, England, July, 1926).

26. Johnston S, Bourne W, Cohen HM, Moots CW. Discussion on the future of anæsthesia: Fostering research in anæsthesia. *Br Med J* 1926;2:775-80. (Presentation: Section of Anæshtetics, British Medical Association Meeting, Nottingham, England, 21st July 1926).

27. Bourne W. On the effects of acetaldehyde, ether peroxide, ethyl mercaptan, ethyl sulphide, and several ketones - di-methyl, ethyl methyl and di-ethyl - when added to anæsthetic ether. *J Pharmacol Exp Ther* 1926;28:409-32.

28. Bourne W. On the effects of acetaldehyde, ether peroxid, ethyl mercaptan, ethyl sulphid and several ketone - di-methyl, ethyl methyl and di-ethyl - when added to anesthetic ether. *Curr Res Anesth Analg* 1927;6:131-40. (With permission: The Journal of Pharmacology and Experimental Therapeutics. Presentation: Scottish Society of Anæsthetists, Associated Anesthetists of the United States and Canada Joint Meeting Glasgow, 6th July, 1926). (Also published in *J Pharmacol Exp Ther* 1926;28:409-32)

29. Bourne W. Anæsthesia in gall bladder surgery. *Can Med Assoc J* 1927;17:1030-3. (Presentation: Canadian Medical Association, Ontario Medical Association, Canadian Society of Anæsthetists Joint Meeting, Toronto, 17th June, 1927).

30. Rosenthal SM, Bourne W. The effects of anesthetics on hepatic function. *Curr Res Anesth Analg* 1928;7:276-9. (Presentation: 6th Annual Congress, Association of Anesthetists of the United States and Canada and International Anesthesia Research Society Joint Meeting, Washington DC, 15th-18th May, 1927).

31. Rosenthal SM, Bourne W. The effects of anesthetics on hepatic function. *JAMA* 1928;90:377-9. (Presentation: Associated Anesthetists of the United States and Canada, Washington D.C., 17th May, 1927). (Also published in *Curr Res Analg Anæsth* 1928;7:276-9)

32. Stehle RL, Bourne W. The effects of morphine and ether on the function of the kidneys. *Arch Intern Med* 1928:42:248-55.

33. Stehle RL, Bourne W. The effects of morphin and ether on the function of the kidneys. *Curr Res Anesth Analg* 1929; 8: 263-8. *(With permission: Archives of Internal Medicine* . Presentation: Eastern Society of Anesthetists and Canadian Society of Anæsthetists Joint Meeting, Boston, Mass, 8th-12th October, 1928). (Also published in *Arch Intern Med* 1928:42:248-55)

1930s

34. Bruger M, Bourne W, Dreyer NB. Effects of avertin on liver function: the rate of secretion and composition of the urine, the reaction, alkali reserve and concentration of the blood and the body temperature. *Am J Surg* 1930;9:82-7.

35. Bourne W, Bruger M, Dreyer NB. The effects of sodium amytal on liver function; the rate of secretion and composition of the urine; the reaction, alkali reserve, and concentration of the blood; and the body temperature. *Surg Gynec Obstet* 1930;51:356-60. (Presentation: Medico-Chirurgical Society, Montreal, 25th April, 1930.

36. Bourne W. What constitutes an efficient anæsthesia service for a hospital. *Bull Amer Coll Surg* 1930;14:30-3. (Presentation: American College of Surgeons, Chicago, 16th October, 1929).

37. Raginsky BB, Bourne W, Bruger M. The effect of avertin upon the circulation. *J Pharmacol Exp Ther* 1931;43:219-31.

38. Bourne W. Abstract: The problem of operating room temperatures (Transactions of 8th Annual Congress of Anesthetists, Chicago, 1929). *Curr Res Anesth Analg* 1931;10:47-8 (Suppl). (Presentation: 8th Annual Congress of Anesthetists, Chicago, 14th October, 1929).

39. Bourne W. The administration of chloroform in obstetrics by nurses. *The Canadian Nurse* 1930;26:585-7.

40. Bourne W, Bruger M, Dreyer NB. The effects of amytal and avertin, separately, on the blood, its reaction, the carbon dioxid combining power, and the concentrabon; on body temperature; on the function of the liver;

and on the rate of secretion and composition of the urine. *Curr Res Anesth Analg* 1931; 10: 85-7. (Presentation: 9th Annual Congress of Anesthetists, International Anesthesia Research Society Joint Meeting with the Eastern Society of Anesthetists, Clinical Congress of Surgeons Week, Hotel Adelphia, Philadelphia, 13th-16th October, 1930).

41. Bourne W, Bruger M, Dreyer NB. The effects of amytal and avertin on the blood. The temperature and the functions of the liver and kidneys. *Can Med Assoc J* 1931;24:384-6. (Presentation: 9th Annual Congress of Anesthetics, Philadelphia, 15th October 1930).

42. Bourne W, Raginsky BB. The effect of avertin upon the normal and impaired liver. *Am J Surg* 1931;14:653-6.

43. Gurd FB, Bourne W. Avertin in surgical anæsthesia . *Can Med Assoc J* 1931;25:587-9. (Presentation: Medico-Chirurgical Society, Montreal, 6th November, 1931).

44. Raginsky BB, Bourne W. The action of ephedrine in avertin anesthesia. *J Pharmacol Exp Ther* 1931;43:209-18.

45. Bourne W. The present status of avertin in anæsthesia. *Can Med Assoc J* 1932;27:515-6. (Presentation: Section of Anæsthetics, Canadian Medical Association Meeting, Toronto, 22nd June, 1932).

46. Bourne W. The effects of anæsthetics on the liver. *BMJ* 1932;2:706-7. (Presentation: Section of Anæsthetics, Centenary Meeting of British Medical Association, London, 1932).

47. Raginsky BB, Bourne W. On several phases of the pharmacology of avertin. *Curr Res Anesth Analg* 1932;11:33-7. (Presentation: 10th Annual Congress of Anesthetists, International Anesthesia Research Society Joint Meeting with Associated Anesthetists of United States and Canada, Eastern Society of Anesthetists and Mid-Western Association of Anesthetists, Clinical Congress of Surgeons' Week, New York, NY, 12th-16th October, 1931).

48. Raginsky BB, Bourne W. Abstract: Pharmacology of avertin (*Curr Res Anesth Analg* 1932;11:33-7). *Br J Anæsth* 1932;9:135.

49. Bourne W. Some phases of the pharmacology of anæsthetics. *Oral Health* 1932;22:563-9. (Presentation: Montreal Dental Club, Montreal, 29th January, 1932).

50. Bourne W. Avertin: a new anæsthetic. *The Canadian Nurse* 1933;29:397-400.

51. Bourne W. Abstract: Present status of avertin in anesthesia (*Can Med Assoc J* 1932; 27: 515-6). *Curr Res Anesth Analg* 1933; 12: 734 (suppl).

52. Bourne W, Raginsky BB. Avertin anesthesia *American Medicine* 1933;39:(4)5-7 and 24.

53. McKim LH, Bourne W. The use of avertin in multiple dressings: effects on the liver. *Can Med Assoc J* 1933;28:149-51. (Presentation: Montreal Medico-Chirurgical Society, 18th November, 1932).

54. Bourne W, Raginsky BB. Avertin anesthesia. *American Medicine* 1933; New Series 28 (v):5-7 and 24.

55. Bourne W, Raginsky BB. Avertin anesthesia. *International Journal of Medicine and Surgery* 1933; 46: 229-32. (Also published in *American Medicine* 1933; New Series 28 (v):5-7 and 24.).

56. Raginsky BB, Bourne W. The oxygen content of blood during nitrous oxid-oxygen anesthesia in man. *Curr Res Anesth Analg* 1934;13:152-5. (Presentation: 12th Annual Congress of Anesthetists, International Anesthesia Research Society Joint Meeting with Associated Anesthetists of United States and Canada, Eastern Society of Anesthetists, Mid-Western Association of Anesthetists and Southern Association of Anesthetists, Clinical Congress of Surgeons Week, Chicago, Ill., 9th-12th October, 1933).

57. Bourne W, O'Shaughnessy PE. Abstract: One thousand avertin anæsthesias. (*Can Med Assoc* J 1934;31:276-84). *Br J Anæsth* 1934; 12: 47-8.

58. Raginsky BB, Bourne W. Cynanosis in nitrous oxide oxygen anæsthesia in man. *Can Med Assoc* J 1934;30:518-22.

59. Bourne W. An estimate of the usefulness of some of the newer anæsthetics in practice. *Can Med Assoc J* 1934;31:44-7. (Presentation: 65th Annual Meeting of Canadian Medical Association, Calgary, 20th June, 1934).

60. Bourne W, O'Shaughnessy PE. One thousand avertin anæsthesias. *Can Med Assoc J* 1934;31:276-84.

61. Raginsky B, Bourne W. Effects of cyclopropane on the normal and impaired liver. *Can Med Assoc J* 1934;31:500-1.

62. Bourne W. Divinyl oxide anæsthesia in obstetrics. *Lancet* 1934;1:566-7. (Presentation: Medico-Chirurgical Society, Montreal, 17th November, 1933).

63. Bourne W. Cyclopropane anæsthesia in obstetrics. *Lancet* 1934; 2: 2-1.

64. Bourne W, Raginsky BB. Vinyl ether (vinesthene) anæsthesia in dogs: effects upon normal and impaired liver. *Br J Anæsth* 1935;12:62-9. (Award: Best essay in *British Journal of Anæsthesia* 1934 Competition).

65. Bourne W, Sparling DW. Some aspects of vinyl ether (vinethene) anesthesia. *Curr Res Anesth Analg* 1935;14:4-7. (Presentation: 13th Annual Congress of Anesthetists, International Anesthesia Research Society Joint Meeting with Associated Anesthetists of United States and Canada, Eastern Society of Anesthetists, Mid-Western Association of Anesthetists, and Boston Society of Anesthetists, Clinical Congress of Surgeons Week Boston Mass., 15th-19th October, 1934). (Also published in *Br J Anæsth* 1935;12:62-9)

66. Bourne W. Abstract: An estimate of the usefulness of avertin in surgical practice (*Can Med Assoc J* 1934;31:44-7). *Curr Res Anesth Analg* 1935;14:76-7 (suppl).

67. Bourne W, Sparling DW. Abstract: Considérations sur l'anesthésie à l'éther divinylique (*Curr Res Anesth Analg* 1935;14:4-7). *Anésthesie Analgésie* 1935;1: 18.

68. Bourne W. Raginsky BB. Abstract: L'anesthésie a l'ether divinylique chez le chien: son action sur le foie sain et malade (*Br J Anæsth* 1935; 12:

62-9). *Anésthesie Analgésie* 1935;1:318.

69. Bourne W. Vinyl ether obstetric anesthesia for general practice. *JAMA* 1935; 105: 2047-51. (Presentation: Section on Obstetrics and Gynecology, 86th Annual Session of American Medical Association, Atlantic City, NJ, 14th June, 1935).

70. Bourne W. Vinyl ether obstetrical anæsthesia for general practice. *Can Med Assoc J* 1935;33:629-32. (Presentation: Section on Obstetrics and Gynecology, 86th Annual Session of American Medical Association, Atlantic City, NJ, 14th June, 1935). (Also published in *JAMA* 1935;105: 2047-51)

71. Bourne W. Avertin anæsthesia for crippled children. *Can Med Assoc J* 1936;5:278-81.

72. Bourne W, O'Shaughnessy PE. The Etherington-Wilson technique in intrathecal segmental analgesia. *Can Med Assoc J* 1936;35:536-49.

73. Anesthetics and liver function. *Am J Surg* 1936;34:486-95.

74. Bourne W, McDowell JF, Whyte JC. Further studies in vinyl ether (vinethene) obstetrical anesthesia: mixtures with ethyl ether: effect on coagulation time of blood. *Curr Res Anesth Analg* 1937;16:46-51. (Presentation: 15th Annual Congress of Anesthetists, International Anesthesia Research Society Joint Meeting with Associated Anesthetists of United States and Canada Eastern Society of Anesthetists, Mid-Western Association of Anesthetists and Southern Association of Anesthetists, Clinical Congress of Surgeons Week Philadelphia, Pa, 19th-23rd October, 1936).

75. Bourne W, Dowell JF, Whyte JC. Nouvelles recherches sur l'éther divinylique (vinéthène) en anesthésie obstétricale. Mélange avec l'éther éthylique: effets sur la coagulation du sang. *Anesthésie Analgésie* 1937;3:136. (Presentation: Congrès intemational d'anesthésie de Philadelphia, 19th-23rd October, 1936).

76. MacPhail FL, Gray HD, Bourne W. Pentothal sodium as a hypnotic in obstetrics. *Can Med Assoc J* 1937;37:471-4.

77. Dworkin S, Bourne W, Raginsky BB. Changes in conditioned responses brought about by anæsthetics and sedatives. *Can Med Assoc J* 1937; 37:136-9.

78. Dworkin S, Raginsky BB, Bourne W. Action of anesthetics and sedatives upon the the inhibited nervous system. *Curr Res Anesth Analg* 1937; 16:238-40. (Presentation: 15th Annual Congress of Anesthetists, International Anesthesia Research Society and Associated Anesthetists of the United States and Canada, Eastern Society of Anesthetists, Mid-Western Association of Anesthetists and Southern Association of Anesthetists, Clinical Congress of Surgeons Week Philadelphia, Pa, 19th-23rd October, 1936).

79. Dworkin S, Bourne W, Raginsky BB. Action des anesthésiques, sédatifs, hynotiques sur les centres nerveux superieurs. *Anesthésie Analgésie* 1937; 3:33549. (Presentation: Prize competition of the Société d'Anesthésie et d'Analgésie 1936). (Awarded honorable mention)

80. MacPhail FL, Gray HRD, Bourne W. Abstract: Pentothal sodium as a hypnotic in obstetrics. (*Can Med Assoc J* 1937;37:471-4) *Br J Anæsth* 1937;15:82-3.

81. Dworkin S, Bourne W, Raginsky BB. Abstract: Changes in conditional responses, due to anæsthetics. (*Can Med Assoc J* 1937;37:136-9). *Br J Anæsth* 1937;15:83.

82. Bourne W. Analgesia and anesthesia in obstetrics: pentothal sodium, cyclopropane and vinyl ether. *NY State J Med* 1937;22:1905-8. (Presentation: Annual Meeting, Medical Society of the State of New York Rochester, 25th May, 1937).

83. Bourne W. Analgesia and anæsthesia in obstetrics: pentothal sodium, cyclopropane and vinyl ether. *Br J Anaesth* 1937;15:1-81. (With permission: *New York State Journal of Medicine*). (Also published in *NY State J Med* 1937;22:1905-8)

84. Bourne W. Abstract: Anesthésiques et fonction hépatique (*Amer J Surg* 1936; 34: 486-95) *Anesthésie Analgésie* 1938;4:121.

85. Bourne W, O'Shaughnessy PE. Abstract: La technique d'Etherington-Wilson dans l'analgésie segmentaire intra-dure-merienne (*Can Med Assoc J* 1936;35:536-40). *Anesthésie Analgésie* 1938;4:130.

86. Bourne W. Abstract: L'anesthésie a l'avertine chez les enfants infirmes (*Can Med Assoc J* 1936;35:278-81). *Anesthésie Analgésie* 1938;4:134.

87. Gurd FB, Vineberg AM, Bourne W. Our experiences in the employment of spinal anesthesia for thoracoplasty. *Journal of Thoracic Surgery* 1938;7:506-11. (Presentation: 20th Annual Meeting of American Association for Thoracic Surgery, Saranac Lake, New York, 3lst May - 2nd June 1937).

88. Bourne W. The perfecting of anæsthesia. *Can Med Assoc J* 1938;39:249-53. (Presentation: McGill Chemical Society, Montreal, 4th February, 1938).

89. Bourne W. Anæsthesia for the Republic of Plato. *Yale Journal of Biology and Medicine* 1938;11:149-60. (Presentation. Seminar, Department of Pharmacology and Toxicology, Yale University School of Medicine, 24th, October, 1938).

90. Bourne W. Fors clavigera in anæsthesia *Can Med Assoc J* 1939;40:524. (Presentation: 69th Annual Meeting of Canadian Medical Association, Halifax, 22nd June, 1938).

91. Bourne W. Anesthesia. *Hospitals* 1939;13 (January):97-8. (Presentation: 21st Annual Hospital Standardization Conference, American College of Surgeons, October 1938).

92. Bourne W. Anesthesia in the hospital. *Hospital Management* 1938;46:39-41. (Presentation: Hospital Standardization Conference of the American College of Surgeons, New York, 20th October, 1938). (Also published in *Hospitals* 1939;13 (January):97-8)

93. Bourne W, Pauly AJ. Thiobarbiturates in obstetrics: Pentothal and thioethamyl. *Can Med Assoc J* 1939;40:437-40.

94. Bourne W. Anesthesia In: A discussion of important questions and

problems pertaining to various phases of hospital administration. (Report of Administrative Panel Round Table Conference. *Bull Amer Surg* 1939; 24: 220-34). *Bull Amer Coll Surg* 1939;24:228-9.

95. Bourne W. Factors determining selection and administration of anesthetics. *Surg Gynecol Obstet* 1939;68:519-26. (Presentation: Symposium on surgical procedures on the handicapped patient, Clinical Congress of the Royal College of Surgeons, New York, 17th-21st October, 1938).

96. Bourne W. Trends in inhalation anesthesia. *Ann Surg* 1939;110:83-4. (Presentation: American Surgical Association, Hot Springs, Virginia, llth-13th May, 1939).

97. Gurd FB, Vineberg AM, Bourne W. Further experiences in the use of spinal anesthesia for thoracoplasty. *Ann Surg* 1939;110:872-7. (Presentation: American Surgical Association, Hot Springs, Virginia 11th-13th May 1939).

1940s

98. *Bourne W. Francis Hoeffer Mc Mechan: an apotheosis. *Curr Res Anesth Analg* 1940;19 i: Pages not given. Article specially included (Jan-Feb 1940). (Presentation: Memorial Address during the 18th Annual Congress of Anesthetists. Philadelphia, 16th-20th October, 1939).

99. Bourne W. Presidential address: Anesthesia in perspective. *Curr Res Anesth Analg* 1940;19:181-3. (Presentation: 18th Annual Congress of Anesthetists, International College of Anesthetists, Joint Meeting with Eastern Society of Anesthetists and Philadelphia County Dental Society, Clinical Congress Congress Surgical Week Philadelphia Pa, 16th-20th October 1939).

100. Bourne W. Choice of anæsthesia in emergency surgery. *The Journal of the Michigan State Medical Society* 1942;41:35-8. (Presentation: 76th Annual Meeting of the Michigan State Medical Society, Grand Rapids, Michigan, 19th September, 1941).

101. Bourne W. De officius in anæsthesia *Journal of the Michigan State Medical Society* 1942;41:129-34. (Presentation: 76th Annual Meeting of the Michigan State Medical Society, Grand Rapids, Michigan, 17th September, 1941).

102. Bourne W. Interdependence of function in anesthesia. *JAMA* 1942;120:997-9. (Presentation: Section on Anesthesiology, 93rd Annual Session of American Medical Association, Atlantic City, NJ, 11th June, 1942).

103. Bourne W. Editorial: Breathing in anesthesia. *Anesthesiology* 1942; 3:204-10.

104. Bourne W, Leigh MD, Inglis NA, Howell GR. Spinal anesthesia for thoracic surgery. *Anesthesiology* 1942;3:272-81.

105. Bourne W. Anæsthesia for the tuberculous patient. *Br J Anæsth* 1942;18:49-59. (Presentation: Meeting of the Section on Tuberculosis, the Montreal Medico-Chirurgical Society, 21st January, 1942).

106. Bourne W. Editorial: Presidential address. *Anesthesiology* 1942;3:448-52. (Presentation: American Society of Anesthetists. Inc. New York, 12th February. 1942).

107. Bourne W. Abstract: Anæsthesia in war circumstances (*Can Med Assoc J* 1942;46:241-5). *Anesthesiology* 1942;3:588-90.

108. Bourne W. Anæsthesia in war circumnstances. *Can Med Assoc J* 1942;46:241-5. (Presentation: Annual Meeting of Massachusetts Medical Society, 22nd May, 1941).

109. Bourne W. Pure ether and impurities: a review. *Anesthesiology* 1946; 7:599-605. (Presentation: Meeting of Anesthesiologists, Mayo Clinic, 24th May, 1945 and Presentation: Medico-Chirurgical Society Meeting, Montreal, 10th May, 1946).

110. Bourne W. The centennium of anæsthesia. *CAMSI Journal* 1946;5: 25-8.

111. Bourne W. Gaseous anæsthetics. Anesthesiology 1947;8:227-35. (Presentation: Morton Centennial, Joint Meeting of American Society of Anesthesiologists, Inc. and New England Society of Anesthesiology, Boston, Mass., 16th October, 1946).

112. Bourne W. Guest editorial: Post-graduate education in anæsthesia. *Virginia Medical Monthly* 1948;75:1-3.

113. Bourne W. At the head of the table. *California Medicine* 1948;69: 425-8. (Presentation: 2nd General Meeting of the 77th Annual Session of California Medical Association, San Francisco, 11th-14th April, 1948).

114. Bourne W. What's new in anesthesia. *California Medicine* 1948;68: 426-8. (Presentation: Panel Discussion, General Meeting, 77th Annual Session of the California Medical Association, San Francisco, Ca, 11th-14th April, 1948).

115. Bourne W. Impressions of the centenary celebrations of anæsthesia in Great Britain. *Anesthesiology* 1948;9:239-50.

116. Bourne W. Impressions of the centenary celebrations of anæsthesia in Great Britain (continued). *Anesthesiology* 1948;9:358-72.

117. Bourne W. Abstract: Guest editorial, post-graduate education in anæsthesia (*Virginia Medical Monthly* 1948;75:1-3). *Anesthesiology* 1948;9:659-60.

118. Bourne W. Wise indifference of the wise in anesthesia. *Am J Obstet Gynecol* 1948; 55: 711-6. (Correction: *Am J Obstet Gynecol* 1948; 55:1075). (Presentation: Annual Meeting of American Association of Obstetricians, Gynecologists and Abdominal Surgeons, Hot Springs, Va, 4th-6th September, 1947).

119. Bourne W. Wise indifference of the wise in anesthesia. *Am J Obstet Gynecol* 1948; 55: 711-6. (Presentation: Annual Meeting of American Association of Obstetricians, Gynecologists and Abdominal Surgeons, Hot Springs, Va, 4th September, 1947). (Also published in the *Transactions of the American Association of Obstetrics and*

Gynecologists and Abdominal Surgeons 1947;58:221-8)

120. Griffith HR, Stephen CR, Cullen WG, Bourne W. Myanesin as a muscle relaxant. *Anesthesiology* 1949;10:61-5.

121. Bourne W. The role of basic sciences in anesthesia. *Curr Res Anesth Analg* 1949;28:288-9. (Presentation: 23rd Annual Congress of Anesthetists Joint Session of International Anesthesia Research Society and International College of Anesthetists, Montreal, Canada, 18th-21st October, 1948).

122. Bourne W. On learning anæsthesia. *Anesthesiology* 1949;10:157-63. (Presentation: Regional Meeting of American Society of Anesthesiologists, Kansas City, Ma, 5th April, 1948).

123. Bourne W. Anæsthesia and the pursuit of learning. *Can Med Assoc J* 1948;59:70-2. (Presentation: Anæsthesia section of Ontario Medical Association Meeting, Kingston, 20th November, 1947). (Also published in *Anesthesiology* 1949;10:157-63)

1950s

124. * Bourne W. Measure and order in a school of anæsthesia. *Asociacion Argentina de Anestesiologia* 1950;22 and 142-51.

125. * Griffith HR, Bourne W. Muscle relaxants. *Asociacion Argentina de Anestesiologia* 1950;385-91.

126. Asquith E, Bourne W, Gilbert RGB. Trichlorethylene - the McGill vaporizer. *Can Med Assoc J* 1950;62:604-5.

127. Griffith HR, Stephen CR, Cullen WG, Bourne W. Abstract: La myanésine pour le relachement musculaire (*Anesthesiology* 1949; 10:61-5). *Anesthésie Analgésie* 1950;7:127.

128. Bourne W. Essentials of an efficient anæsthetic service. *Canadian Hospital* 1950;27:32-3 and 52. (Presentation: Sectional Meeting of American College of Surgeons, Montreal, 20th March, 1950).

129. Bourne W. Editorial: Latin-American Anesthesia. *Curr Res Anesth Analg* 1951;30:120.

130. Bourne W. Recent advances in anesthesia. *Curr Res Anesth Analg* 1951;30:241-9. (Presentation: 25th Annual Congress of Anesthetists Joint Session of International Anesthesia Research Society and International College of Anesthetists, Miami Beach, Fla., 30th October - November 2nd, 1950 and Presentation: Sectional Meeting of American College of Surgeons, Montreal, Canada, 21st March, 1950).

131. Bourne W, Gilbert RGB. Anesthesia. *Annual Review of Medicine* 1952; 3:157-74.

132. Bourne W. Editorial: Significant form in anæsthesia. *Anesthesiology* 1955;16:454-63. (Presentation: Meeting of New England Society of Anesthesiologists, Hanover, New Hampshire, 8th October, 1954).

133. Hosein EA, Stachiewicz E, Bourne W, Denstedt OF. The influence of nitrous oxide on the metabolic activity of brain tissue. *Anesthesiology* 1955;16:708-15. (Presentation: Annual Meeting, Armerican Society of Anesthesiologists, Inc., Cincinnati Ohio, 27th October, 1954).

134. Bourne W. *Mysterious Waters to Guard: Essays and Addresses on Anæsthesia*. Blackwell Scientific Publications, Oxford, 1955.

135. Bourne W: Foreword to *Elements of Pædiatric Anesthesia* by CR Stephen, Ryerson Press, Toronto, 1955. (This book was reviewed in *Can J Anæsth* 1955;2:296 by Code Smith).

136. Bourne W. Editorial: The address given by Dr. Wesley Bourne on the occasion of the annual dinner of the Canadian Anæsthetists' Society at Toronto, June 21, 1955. *Can Anæsth Soc J* 1955;2:297-300. (Presentation: Annual Meeting, Canadian Anæsthetists' Society, Toronto, June 21st 1955).

137.** Bourne W. On the duties of the anæsthesiologist as a physician. *Curr Res Anesth Analg* 1956;35:115-22. (Presentation: 8th Postgraduate Refresher Course in Anesthesiology, University of Kansas, 11th April, 1955).

138. Bourne W. The effects of excess carbon dioxide (hypercapnia) during anæsthesia; (A review). *Curr Res Anesth Analg* 1956;35:274-284. (Presentation: 8th Annual Postgraduate Refresher Course in Anesthesiology, University of Kansas, 13th April, 1955).

* These articles were reproduced in *Mysterious Waters to Guard*, but not located in the original.

** This article was quoted in Martin et al. *Anesth Analg* 1991;73:221-5 and Fine. *Anesth Analg* 1992;74:327.

VIII

Selected Quotations

In compiling this biography, Wesley Bourne's publications have been used as the undisputed record of his career activities. Therefore, it has been possible to discuss the state of Canadian anæsthesia, his family life, and the Montreal milieu in which he lived and worked, with the confidence that comes from the authority of the written word. Although Wesley Bourne's papers have been a source of considerable practical value, they also deserve to be read for "Fun." The following quotations have been selected, fairly arbitrarily, as representative of his writing on clinical practice, research, administration and philosophical matters. All are interesting, not so much for the subject to hand, but as illustrations of Wesley Bourne's style and depth of knowledge. Where definitions or explanations were needed, the *Shorter Oxford English Dictionary*[1], *Encyclopædia Britannica*[2] or Plato's *Republic*[3] were consulted.

On clinical practice

1. "In those cases where vomiting is a troublesome symptom, it is found advisable to wash out the stomach, and where the contents of the small bowel are liable to continue to regurgitate, the stomach tube may be left in for futher emptying and lavage."

   (*Can Med Assoc J* 1924;14:835-6).

2. "We have several other means of producing anæsthesia in cocaine and its derivatives, procaine, nitrous oxide, the barbiturates and tribromethanol. The proper attitude being to suit the drug to the case in question, considering the necessities of that which has to be done. There may never be any panacea in anæsthesia."

   (*Oral Health* 1932;22:563-9).

---

[1] Onions CT (Ed). *The Shorter Oxford English Dictionary on Historical Principles*, 3rd ed. Oxford: The Clarendon Press, 1972.

[2] Goetz PW (Ed). *The New Encyclopædia Britannica*, 15th ed. Chicago, London, Toronto: Encyclopædia Britannica Inc., 1768.

[3] Lee D (Translator). Plato, *The Republic*, 2nd ed. London, Toronto: Penguin Books, Ltd., 1972.

3. "It is an old problem, that of the relief of pain in obstetrics, and its solutions are still the subject of great controversy."

(*Br J Anæsth* 1937;15:1-8. & *New York State Journal of Medicine* 1937;37:905-8).

On research

1. "Of the fifteen cases here reported, eleven show a definite increased phophorus excretion as a consequence of the anesthesia. .....Possibly, the greater excretion of phosphorus following the anesthetic is due to a period of oliguria accompanying the anesthetic...same effect by nitrous oxide, ether and chloroform."

(*JAMA* 1924;83:117-8).

2. "When morphine is administered as a preliminary to etherization a marked excretion of phosphorus occurs as soon as the ether is begun. This is attributed to an action of the morphine upon the liver which renders it incapable of retaining phosphorus. It is suggested that the low alkali reserve and increased acidity of the blood in ether anesthesia is due to the discharge of phosphoric acid from the muscles."

(*J Biol Chem* 1924;60:17-29).

3. "Research zeal has been particularly keen in recent times, and it is common knowledge that considerable light has been shown on some of our propositions.....advances in obstetrical anesthesia, in insufflation methods, in the many methods of administering anesthetics generally."

(*Br Med J* 1926;2:775-80).

4. "Brief periods of chloroform anesthesia are sufficient to produce immediate and delayed toxic effects on the liver; half an hour of chloroform causes injury that requires eight days for functional recovery, while two hours of anesthesia requires six weeks to return to normal."

(*Curr Res Anesth Analg* 1928;7:276-9).

5. "The effects of ether and morphine acting separately and concomitantly on the secretion of water, urea and chlorides by the kidneys have been studied....in general, when each of these substances acts alone kidney activity is diminished, it is shown that when they act concomitantly the

amount of secretion is greater than it is with ether alone."
(*Archives of Internal Medicine* 1928;42:248-55. & *Curr Res Anesth Analg* 1929;8:263-8).

6. "Experiments on dogs and observations in man are described which show that rectal anæsthesia with avertin (tribromethanol) may be interrupted or considerably shortened by the administration of ephedrine. This property of ephedrine is of value clinically in overcoming too profound avertin anesthesia."
(*J Pharmacol Exp Therap* 1931;43:209-18).

7. "The inchoactive studies of Leake and Chen were done with impure material."
(*Curr Res Anesth Analg* 1935;14:4-7)

On administration

1. "In my opinion the department of anæsthesia in any large hospital is so important to the efficient work and prestige of that hospital to imply the demand that its chief, the senior anæsthetist, should be accorded a place on the medical board with rights equal to those of all the other members.... Such a man must posssess considerable ability, must be a student himself and keep up to date, not to mention the personal qualities necessary for good will among the members of the staff."
(*Bull Amer Coll Surg* 1930;14:30-3).

2. "When the hospital personnel is such that the services of a competent anesthetist are momentarily available, then each member of the anesthesia staff will be a graduate in medicine; this staff will consist of a director, assistant director, enough associate anesthetists for the surgical requirements, a resident anesthetist, and as many interne anesthetists as the work necessitates. If the hospital is connected with a medical school, there will be a system of fellowships, as exemplified by the University of Wisconsin, partly taking the place of associate and interne anesthetists.
(*Bull Amer Coll Surg* 1939;24:220-34).

3. "Nine years ago....it was my privilege to lead the discussion on anesthesia. .....Not nearly enough has been done, however, and it seems a pity that

the American College of Surgeons should summon these gatherings so painstakingly year by year, to enunciate reiteratively the principles of the practice of anesthesia with so little heeding and such dilatory results. But then all human behavior is woefully wanting. Plato's Republic* is far in the seeking!"

(*Hospitals* 1939;13 (January):97-8).

[*Plato's Republic: "The Republic" is the ideal State envisaged by Plato, the second of the three great Greek philosophers, who followed Socrates and preceded Aristotle. His underlying concern is ethical and a vision of justice based on what is good. He saw a harmonious society as one in which all parts function well and do not interfere with each other. This translated into a tripartite scheme of "state order" depending on the three lives of man as a philosopher (with wisdom, the statesmen), a votary of enjoyment (seeking gratification, the population at large) and a man of action (practical, the army). When it came to training intellectuals, he saw a scheme whereby they would learn the basic knowledge in their first ten years and then apply this in the next five years by dialectic learning, or the art of conversation. By conversation, he meant the ability to pose and answer questions about the essence of things and to frame all scientific knowledge securely in basic principles. Out of all this, came "the good", or the enlightenmnt which suddenly dawns as the goal is close to being achieved].

4. "Nevertheless, it is not in the province of the nurse to familiarize herself too much with the meticulous details that go along with the use of these substances."

(*The Canadian Nurse* 1930;26:585-7).

A supportive comment in the discussion on Wesley Bourne's presentation, made by Dr. I. Hird:

> With the interest of the patient, surgeon and hospital in mind, I do not hesitate to say that I doubt the wisdom of the present tendency to employ lay anæsthetists, and it is my profound belief that the system of salaried non-medical anæshtetists is not only contrary to the medical practice act and professional ethics but it will surely result in the degeneration of the art of anæsthesia and greatly hinder all advancement in this line of medical research.

(*Bull Amer Coll Surg* 1930;14:30-3).

At the fourth annual Congress of Anesthetists with the Associated Anesthetists of the United States and Canada and International Anæsthesia Research Society joint meeting in Atlantic City, Wesley Bourne's presidential address verged, at times, on the condescending:

> You have done more than confer an honor on me, for with your customary generosity you have given preference to an associate of McGill University and a member of the Canadian Anæsthetists' Society, in other words, to a Canadian. It is by no means the first occasion on which you have bestowed your best decorations on others than those of your own great country.
>
> (*Curr Res Anesth Analg* 1925;4:259-66).

It was equalled by Dr. F.E. Shipway's introduction at the Royal Society of Medicine meeting in the following year:

> Dr Shipway said that he felt that the United States had great traditions to live up to in anæsthesia, and he could not help thinking that by their presence here, the American anæsthetists showed they were conscious of the debt they owed to their forerunners in the past, and that they were anxious to live up to the high standard which has been set them.
>
> (*Proc Roy Soc Med* 1926;19, Section of Anæsthesia:49-51).

On philosophical matters

1. "Fear may lead to phantasmagoria of excruciating incident to the patient going under an anesthetic, something like the wild ideas of [?] in the land of dreams depicted by Edgar Allen Poe in some of his weird but beautifully written tales of mystery and imagination. .....The anesthetist does well to take upon himself the role of *μονσικς*, that is, as Plato meant it to be in the broader sense."
(*Ann Surg* 1939;110;830-4).

2. It is with the hormone of the Graafian follicle that we are at present interested......In conclusion it would seem that we are on the eve of having at once a boon in the hands of the conscientious, and a curse with profligacy and panderism.
(*Can Med Assoc J* 1925;15:171-3).

3. There is no dilettantism about Waters. Had Carlyle known him, he would have mentioned him as one of the Heroes in his "Hero-Worship."* This, I shall say: he has emulated the sculptor, Φετδίας, who while construction the Athene in the Acropolis carved his own face in the centre of her shield, and connected it by an imperceptible artifice with the statue, so that the one became inseparable from the other. Throughout the theme of anæsthesia one finds many instances of serendipity, some associated with chance and others with sagacity.
(*Can Med Assoc J* 1938;39:249-53).

[*"**Hero-Worship**": Thomas Carlyle's 1841 publication *On Heroes, Hero-Worship, and the Heroic in History*. One of the major works of this Calvanistic British historian and essayist (1795-1881). It showed his reverence for strength, especially when this was to achieve a God-given mission. He saw his "Hero" as the divinity (pagan myths), prophet (Muhammad), poet (Dante and Shakespeare), priest (Luther and Knox), man of letters (Johnson and Burns), and king (Cromwell and Napoleon). Carlyle's view of life in the West Indies may lend a clue to the attitudes prevalent in those islands when Wesley Bourne was growing up in Barbados. The governor had brutally put down an uprising in 1865, and Carlyle rallied to his support with the words: "Saving the West Indies and hanging one incendiary mulatto, well worth the gallows, if I can judge."]

4. While Plato wished to rise to a knowledge of the Supreme Idea through the realization of the lower ideas, and showed that these contain the essence of things, he pointed out that it is the object of science completely to disclose the attributes of all entities, the idea of good being the keystone of all rational investigation ....Anyone contemplating a surgical operation is subject to some degree of fear, from mild apprehension to extreme dread. Out of it may come excruciating phantasmagoria during the period of going under an anæsthetic, and such spectres are so realistic that severe shock may ensue, the end-result of which nobody can foretell......In conclusion, while regretting the postponement of Plato's Republic, let us so cultivate our science that we may have anæsthesia fit for this Republic, so desperately needed, so woefully forgotten.
(*Yale Journal of Biology and Medicine* 1938;11:149-60).

5. There is not less wit nor less invention in applying rightly a thought one finds in a book than in being the first author of that thought.

Thus wrote Peter Bayle in 1696, giving many illustrious examples and likening the opposition to a foolish affectation never to quote anybody, and to fetch everything from home; like that Aelian Hippias who merrily boasted all he had about him was his own handiwork. Emerson too, has said that by necessity, by proclivity, and by delight we all quote. Thus it is that I do not hesitate to borrow from Ruskin his *Fors Clavigera*,* and copy his meanings of these words out of a desire to present some observations in a desultory and accidental manner.

(*Can Med Assoc J* 1939;40:52-4).

[***Fors Clavigera:** The translation from the Latin is explicit enough: fors (force, fortune, fortitude), clava (club, key, rudder) and gero (I carry, gesture, jest). The application to anæsthesia is in defining the strength to the anæsthetist in terms of telling of "the fortitude of the workers in the field" and making "a few cogent rules in ordering relevant fortunes". Thus, the justification for the use of Ruskin's title for this discourse on giving good clinical anæsthesia, backed by scientific understanding. John Ruskin (1819-1900), was a English writer, critic and artist who championed the Gothic Revival in architecture. In 1869, he was elected to be first Slade Professor of Fine Art at Oxford. He was an orginal thinker and wanted to identify with a different intellectual class. Accordingly, he wrote letters to the working class, the second of which was *Fors Clavigera* based on his organization of the Company of St. George (founded in 1871, with his endowment of £10,000, in anticipation that each "companion" would give one tenth of his income, as Ruskin did, to this cause).]

In conclusion

"Although in the truly etymological sense anæsthetic and aesthetic are antithetic, and it may seem paradoxical to speak of them in the same breath, yet there is much of the one in the other and æsthetic tendencies are not uncommon to anæsthesia ....continue to follow and emulate the precepts of Anaxagoras, the most illustrious of the early scientists, who influenced Thucydides to incarnate the modern spirit and to lay the foundation of serious historical writing, who influenced Hippocrates to emancipate medicine from religion and to transfer an empirical craft into a scientific tool.

(*Curr Res Anesth Analg* 1940;19:181-3).

IX

LEGACY

The 50th Anniversary of the founding of the McGill Department of Anesthesia is a time to reflect on the past and look to the future. Wesley Bourne, the founding chairman, had the knowledge, enthusiasm, leadership and drive needed to initiate change. He was ahead of his times, but a man of his day. He did what was needed to get things done, and stimulated others to follow his lead. Perhaps, better than anyone, he understood the needs of the specialty and incorporated these thoughts into his presidential address to the American Society of Anesthesiologists' Meeting in New York in 1942:

> ...the more I contemplate this our institution, the more convinced I am that it is sound at heart, and that its strength is the strength of youth. As time goes on, my successors will, I hope, be able to boast of glorious achievement; they will be able to vindicate that boast by citing a long list of eminent men, great masters of experimental science, great artists in clinical procedure. They will, I hope, mention with high honour some of my young friends who now hear me; and they will, I also hope, be able to add that their talents and learning were not wasted on selfish or ignoble objects, but were applied to the service of humanity...As we regard all this to be the imperatively pressing problem of the present in anæsthesia, let us seriously consider approaching our authorities, respectfully, with suggestions for amending the teaching of anæsthesia and for a full application of good anæsthesia during war circumstances.... Henry James has said "There's nothing grotesque in a pure ambition, or in a life devoted to it!"

The prophetic cogency of these words is even greater in hindsight, as Wesley Bourne was only a few years short of achieving his own vision: the establishment of the first autonomous anæsthesia department in Canada at McGill. It is valuable to reflect on his "contemplations," with the knowledge of the history of that embryonic department which has since unfolded, and to be aware that they remain apt, even half a century later.

Wesley Bourne's students have made their own names in anæsthesia, met the challenges of innovative drugs and techniques, contributed to scientific advances and taught another generation of anæsthetists. None attests to Wesley Bourne's influence in the intervening years, between the founding of the McGill department and the uncertainties of the next millenium, better than Dr. Jean T. Hugill, retired staff anæsthetist from Vancouver. She writes in December, 1995 with the knowledge that her views represent those of many Canadian anæsthetists:

> My memory of Dr. Wesley Bourne, whom I knew while on the McGill diploma course, was that of an outstanding anæsthetist of our time.
>
> He was an eloquent speaker and his knowledge of the great philosophers and medical pioneers was phenomenal. He was one of the early researchers in the pharmacology and physiology of anæsthetic drugs, especially the effects on the liver. He was fearless and vigilant in using new techniques such as high spinals to improve the anæsthetic for the patient. He was an excellent teacher and passed on to his students many important tricks and methods in the art of anæsthesia.
>
> He had a far-sighted vision and enthusiasm for the specialty—ahead of his time—which resulted in the establishment of the three-year diploma course at McGill, and the production of well-trained anæsthetists. His outstanding guidance to the advancement of anæsthesia is a landmark in the history of the specialty.
>
> As Dr. Bourne quoted, Aeschylus did say, 'It is ever a joy for the old to learn,' he gave his students the enthusiasm and stimulation to carry on and improve the standard of anæsthesia.

The evolution of anæsthetic practice in the fifty years since Wesley Bourne's appointment has resulted in remarkably safe clinical anæsthesia, high academic standards and involvement of anæsthetists in patient care outside of the operating room. The specialty has achieved the same recognition as other branches of medicine and national and international societies of anæsthesia are flourishing. Although the growth of anæsthetic literature has resulted in nearly one hundred anæsthetic journals in circulation, the importance of these numbers may be over-emphasized and the need for such an increase in publications, doubted[1]. McGill has remained pre-eminent in all aspects of these developments.

---

[1] Greene, N.N. "Anesthesiology journals, 1992." *Anesth Analg*, 1992;74:116-20)

The conflicting interests of university academic anæsthetists and practitioner groups has never been satisfactorily resolved. The problems of financial and political justice which faced Wesley Bourne when he established his academic department, at the same time as he organized clinical service and community education, may, to differing degrees, recur throughout history. Dramatic readjustments had to be made when state medicine, "Medicare", became law in the province of Quebec on 1st November, 1970. In general, the contractual provisions were acceptable to general practitioners, but less so to specialists. Strike action replaced negotiation and the government response, of compulsory return to work under Bill 41, was extremely divisive. Fears were expressed that incomes would decrease by as much as forty percent and that doctors would leave the province. These events were overshadowed by the murder of Pierre Laporte by the Front de Libération du Québec on 17th October, 1970, and physicians embarked on the road towards gradual acceptance of "Medicare". Surgeons resisted the equal recognition afforded to anæsthetists and the proper deployment of anciliary help for the anæsthetist has been controversial. The fact that anæsthetists were accepted as equal to other specialists in these negotiations was due, in large measure, to Wesley Bourne's foresight. As costs of providing medical care in Canada stress the resources of the health care system[2], and solutions are sought to the reorganization of medical schools[3], lessons may be learned by reading Wesley Bourne's publications and applying them to changing cicumstances.

After Wesley Bourne's death, annual memorial lectures in his name were begun. They were introduced initially in May 1965 as part of the Refresher Course. Infrequently, two lectures were given in the same year, and in 1971, the civil unrest in Montreal with the imposition of the restrictions of the War Measures Act, necessitated cancellation of these lectures. Once established, the Wesley Bourne memorial lectures were taken out of the refresher course programme and now take place in September, as the first of the evening lecture of the continuing medical education lecture series for the academic year. This programme has many of the features of the meetings which originated in those gatherings in the Ciba building. The presence of Wesley Bourne's family at the lectures, and at the dinner which follows, has been a constant feature of these

---

[2] Duncan, P.G. "Anesthesia in Canada's health care system." *J Clin Anesth*, 1992;4:52-62.

[3] Perreault, L. "Editorial. Montreal schools of medicine: preparing for the 21st century." *Contemporary Anæsthesia*, April/May 1994;2.

occasions, and serving to maintain strong links with the past for the incoming generations of anæsthetists. Over the years, the distinguished invited Wesley Bourne lecturers, with a formidable list of accomplishments, and their chosen presentations, have reflected the scholarly and philosophical excellence which Wesley Bourne appreciated:

WESLEY BOURNE MEMORIAL LECTURES

1965	E. Manny Papper	*The selection and management of anæsthesia in patients with heart disease.*
1966	J.E. Eckenhoff	*Anæsthesia and systemic function.*
1966	J. Gordon Robson	*Control of respiration.*
1967	John F. Nunn	*Hypoxia.*
1968	Ronald A. Millar	*Role of the sympathetic nervous system in the cardiovascular response to anæsthesia.*
1969	H.H. Bendixen	*The ventilation requirements.*
1970	R. Dery	*Observation on hyperventilation.*
1971	CANCELLED	
1972	J.P. Bunker	*Anæsthesia as a neurologic syndrome.*
1973	W.K. Hamilton	*Toxicity testing - 1973.*
1974	Leroy D. Vandam	*How to learn about anæsthetics by giving anæsthesia - the transplant experience.*
1975	C.P. Larson Jr.	*Change in anæsthetic practices.*
1976	Thomas F. Hornbein	*Highpoxia: man at altitude.*
1977	R.G.B. Gilbert	*A tribute to Wesley Bourne.*
1977	Nicholas M. Greene	*The influence of anæsthesia on the development of surgery, 1846-1900.*
1978	H. Churchill-Davidson	*Anæsthesia - the way ahead.*
1979	Myron B. Laver	*Anæsthesia and coronary artery disease: preconceptions and misconceptions.*
1980	Philip R. Bromage	*Two faces of deafferentation.*
1981	Marcel Boulanger	*Anæsthesia: a difficult dialogue, or the spectre of Antigone.*
1982	John Wade	*Perinatal anæsthesia.*
1983	Alan W. Conn	*Recent advances in fresh water drowning.*
1984	Gertie Marx	*The evolution of obstetrical anæsthesia.*
1985	C. Ronald Stephen	*The greying of America - a medical challenge.*
1986	M. Keith Sykes	*New techniques of respiratory support.*

1987	Bryan Marshall	*The pulmonary circulation during anæsthesia.*
1988	J. Milic Emili	*Flow resistance of the lung and chest wall in anæsthetized humans.*
1989	Margaret Somerville	*Anæsthetists: communicating with the living and the dead.*
1990	John D. Michenfelder	*Seizures, serendipity, science, sham and satisfaction.*
1991	Paul G. Barash	*Cocaine: the Inca's curse or medical miracle?*
1992	J. Earl Wynands	*Contribution of anæsthesia to the development of cardiac surgery. Canadians were there!*
1993	Pierre Foëx	*Silent myocardial ischæmia: a threat to the surgical patient.*
1994	Robert K. Stoelting	*Changing clinical perspectives in anæsthesia practice.*
1995	Frank M. James III	*Lessons learned from obstetric anæsthesia.*
1996	Sebastien Reiz	*The value of additional cardiac testing before vascular surgery.*

The Wesley Bourne memorial lecture subjects covered landmark developments in anæsthesia and the speakers list reads as a *Who's Who* of international anæsthesia. Professor Gordon Robson, who was the Wellcome research professor at McGill (1956-64) returned from England to give the third. He received a DSc degree from McGill in 1984, and in 1987 was admitted as an honorary fellow of the Royal College of Physicians and Surgeons of Canada at a convocation in Winnipeg. He was knighted and, as Sir Gordon, has been the president of the Royal Society of Medicine, master of the Hunterian Institute of the Royal College of Surgery and professor emeritus, University of London, England: a distinguished colleague and friend of McGill. The career of Professor Leroy Vandam, Harvard, stretched from the era of flammable anæsthetics and the first enthusiastic use of curare, to the new nonflammable anæsthetic vapours and synthetic relaxants, earning him recognition as a teacher and the Horace Wells Award.

Dr. R.B.G. Gilbert, a former chairman of the McGill department, as one of his few remaining colleagues, paid tribute to Wesley Bourne and provided an unique perspective of the man. Later, Dr. Philip R. Bromage, who became chairman from 1970 and was recognized as a leading authority on epidural analgesia in obstetrics, spoke eloquently on his topic. Perhaps, one of the lectures which would have delighted Wesley Bourne most was that of Professor Marcel Boulanger, a Laval graduate who practised in rural Quebec before joining the Université de Montréal, where he was the chairman of the anæsthesia department. His philosophical approach to anæsthesia, his *Spectre of Antigone* so closely mirrored the thinking of Wesley Bourne.

Dr. C. Ronald Stephen, the first memorial lecturer to be born in Montreal, had been a resident in the early McGill training programme. After becoming chief of the departments of anæsthesia at the Neurological Institute and Montreal Children's Hospital, he moved to Duke University in North Carolina, and Washington University in St. Louis, as chairman, instituting residency programmes in both units. Others who were more remote from Wesley Bourne's times, but equally prestigious within the specialty continue the theme. Sir M. Keith Sykes, Nuffield Professor of Anæsthesia, Oxford, England, Professor Bryan Marshall, Horatio Wood Professor, University of Pennsylvania, and Professor Robert K. Stoelting of Iowa. Some lecturers belong to closely related disciplines, which bear greatly on the practice of anæsthesia: Professor J. Milic Emili, professor of experimental medicine and director of the Meakins Christie Respiratory Research Laboratory at McGill, and Professor Margaret Somerville, Gale Professor of Law and director of the Centre for Medicine, Ethics and Law at McGill.

Leadership of McGill's Department of Anesthesia has passed through the capable hands of six Chairmen and two who held acting positions: Wesley Bourne (1945-50), Harold R. Griffith (1950-57), Richard G.B. Gilbert (1957-70), Philip R. Bromage (1970-76), Thomas J. McCaughey (Acting 1976-77), John W. Sandison (1977-85), David R. Bevan (1985-91), Gordon S. Fox (Acting 1992-94) and Francesco Carli (from 1994). The special expertise, styles and immediate objectives of these successive Chairmen may have varied, but all have been committed to the goals set by Wesley Bourne: to encourage and promote excellence in clinical service, teaching and research in anæsthesia. When the University decided to discontinue the use of the diphthong in the late 1980s, the official designation of the department changed from "Anæsthesia" to "Anesthesia."

Close ties with his French Canadian colleagues were important to Wesley Bourne and he was recognized for the collegial associations which he fostered. Interactions between these groups has steadily increased, with representation of both groups at present on the teaching staff of the McGill hospitals. In May, 1962, Drs. Griffith and Gilbert proposed and seconded motions to the Council of the Canadian Anæsthetists' Society that the society publications should be bilingual. This resolution was welcomed and over the next few years was gradually implemented. The family of Wesley Bourne had kept the portrait which was given to him by French Canadian anæsthetists in 1950, and they presented this to the McGill Department of Anesthesia on 12th January, 1989. A ceremony was held in the Dean's office at which Dr. Bourne's sons, Robert (a gastroenterologist), John (a businessman) and his nephew, Hilary (an obstetrician) presented the portrait to the department's chairman, Dr. David R. Bevan. Dean Cruess accepted the portrait on behalf of the University and a number of faculty attended. This portrait now hangs in the McGill Department of Anesthesia, alongside that of Dr. Harold R. Griffith.

The establishment of two endowed chairs in memory of these important founders of the department has had a major impact on the directions which the department would follow, by assuring that funding is provided for academic pursuits in the future. Dr. Bourne's family had been very active in giving continued support to the department's activities and been a constant presence at the annual memorial lectures. In the 1970s, Mr. Sidney Dawes, the father of Mrs. John Bourne, and a Montreal businessman and philanthropist, established the "Salta Benevolent Fund" which had supported worthy causes in the city. Through the generosity of Salta Benevolent Fund, the Wesley Bourne Chair of Anesthesia was created to be held by successive chairs of the McGill department, who hold the title of Wesley Bourne Professor of Anesthesia. This was effective on 1st January, 1990 and was announced in the McGill *Reporter* on 17th January, and the Montreal *Gazette* on 3rd February, 1990. The first person named to hold the Chair was Dr. David R. Bevan[4], then chairman of the University department.

Two years later, the Harold Griffith Professorship was created through donations and University funding, with the appointment to be held by an eminent researcher. The first in this line was Dr. François Donati, who had grown up

---

[4] Serendipidously, the translation of *Plato, The Republic* used for reference while reading Wesley Bourne's publications, was translated by Sir Desmond Lee, a Cambridge graduate who was headmaster at Clifton College, Bristol, England (1948-54) when David Bevan entered that school as a student.

in Quebec and studied at McGill. He became internationally recognized for his investigations into neuromuscular blocking agents, a subject pioneered by Harold Griffith fifty years earlier, with the introduction of curare into clinical practice in 1942. Dr. Donati held this position from 1992, until he moved to the chairmanship of the University of Montreal department two years later, setting a high standard for future encumbents to follow.

Wesley Bourne's original society emblem was recently reinterpreted by a Toronto artist, Linda Montgomery, to commemorate the fiftieth anniversary of the Canadian Anæsthetists' Society. This oil painting, titled "Hypnos" was unveiled at the 49th annual meeting in Toronto on 8th June, 1992. The artist took her inspiration from the original emblem to produce a painting that is a composite of a number of symbolic figures. The main subject represents a patient during anæsthesia, surrounded by blue birds (anæsthetists bringing sleep), poppies (agents of sleep), a hand close to the heart (caring), shades of blue (representative of tranquility and the darkness of the cave), shooting star (injection needle) and the thistles (awakening). This modern interpretation has stimulated considerable interest, while provoking further consideration of the meaning of the society's enduring emblem.

Contemporary anæsthetists sometimes quote the principles which Wesley Bourne taught to clarify issues in medical ethical decision-making. His thirty-five year old quotation[5], "The patient is not a problem; he is a person—with a problem" was used in 1991[6] and 1992[7] to argue the merits of orders of advance directives not to resuscitate patients. In 1940 Wesley Bourne anticipated that anæsthetists may be faced with the need to provide assistance in hastening deaths[8]. He wrote "In perspective then, I see the time coming when we shall practice euthanasia and cremation as long ago suggested by Sir Thomas More; when we shall agree with Sir Thomas Browne that 'Themistocles, that slew his soldier in his sleep, was a merciful executioner, 'tis a kind of punishment the mildness of no laws hath invented.'" Thus, the importance of knowing the

---

[5] Bourne, W. "On the duties of the anesthesiologist as a physician." *Curr Res Anesth Analg* 1956;33:115-22.

[6] Martin, R.L., Soifer, B.E., Stevens, W.C. "Ethical issues in anesthesia: the management of the do-not-resuscitate patient." *Anesth Analg* 1991;73:221-5.

[7] Fine, P.G. "Anesthesiology and the discipline of medical ethics: challenges and opportunities." *Anesth Analg* 1992;74:327-8.

[8] Bourne, W. "Anesthesia in perspective." *Curr Res Anesth Analg* 1940;19:181-3.

history of our specialty is becoming evident.

Others may rightfully claim to have administered anæsthetics in Canada before Wesley Bourne and, indisputably, some made major contributions to Canadian anæsthesia. However, in retrospect few would contest Wesley Bourne's right to the title of "The Quinessential Canadian Anæsthetist" as his life has unfolded in this book. Wesley Bourne's legacy is more than his clinical and academic achievements or his model of teaching which is still followed. It is his indelible and individual contribution to the increasing professionalism in anæsthesia which the contemporary McGill Department, Canadian and international anæsthesia exemplify. His stubborn recognition that research and publication will always be important, despite escalating pressures to provide service at lower cost, persists. By these criteria he is, indeed, the quintessential Canadian anæsthetist. These collective memories of Wesley Bourne show him as unusually gifted and dedicated, but with a special quality which allowed him to understand and communicate with those following in his path. The analogy that he was a "Builder of Bridges" to the future generations, used by Frank McMechan as Wesley Bourne embarked on this incredible career, has never been bettered and should not be forgotten. New challenges face contemporary anæsthetists. The present needs to flourish in the knowledge of the past. The future should be shaped by history. Make history that bridges to the future.

X

MILESTONES (1886-1965)

Wesley Bourne MD CM, MSc, FRCP(C), FICA, DA, FACA, FFARCS

1886	Born, 24th April, 1886, Barbados
1907	Enrolled, McGill Faculty of Medicine, 1911
	Graduated, MD CM, McGill (1st in anatomy)
1911-12	Internship, Royal Victoria Hospital, Montreal
1912	Medical officer to CPR in West.
1913	Internship, surgery - anaesthesia, Montreal hospitals
	Married Sara Beatrice McGillis, 29th November, 1913
	Private anaesthetic practice
	Demonstrator in pharmacology.
1914-18	Captain, RCAMC.
1916	James Douglas born.
1918	John Gilbert born.
1920	Canadian Society of Anaesthetists (CSA) formed
	Listed in first directory of North American anaesthetists
1921	Barbara Jean (Mrs. Z.H. Krupski) born
1921-45	Lecturer in pharmacology, McGill
1922	Member, Research Committee, NARS
1922	MSc thesis *"Heat regulation and water exchange and ether"*
1925	Robert Henry born
1924-5	Secretary, Associated Anesthetists of United States.
1925	Silver loving cup and scrolls of recognition presentation by CSA
1925	President, IARS (first term of office)
1926	Silver loving cup presentation by IARS
1927-8	CSA disbanded
	CMA anaesthetic section formed
1929	Founder member, Anaesthetists' Travel Club.
1931	FRCP(C), only anaesthetist until 1951
1932	Vice-president, CMA section of anaesthesia
1934	*British Journal of Anaesthesia* essay prize
1935	First Henry Hill Hickman Medal, RSM, England
1938	DA, RCS England
1938	FICA
1939	Hon. Research President, IARS/ICA
1939-45	Hon. Lt. Col. RCAMC, consultant to Canadian armed forces

1940	President, IARS (second term).
1941	Great Triumvirate (Bourne, Griffith, Leigh)
	Wartime postgraduate training in anaeshtesia
1941	President-elect, ASA
1942	President, ASA
	RCPS(C) certification in anaesthesia introduced
1943	Canadian Anaesthetists' Society (CAS) established
1945	McGill Department of Anaesthesia founded
	First Chairman, McGill Department of Anaesthesia
1946	Assistant professor, McGill
1747	Honorary fellow, American Medical Association
1948	FFARCS, Royal College of Surgeons of Great Britain and Ireland
	Associate professor, McGill
1949	Professor, McGill
1950	Portrait presentation by Quebec anaesthetists
1950	Retired from university appointment, 31st May
1952	Conséiller Technique de Centre d'Anesthésiologie de Paris, WHO
	Academy of Anesthesiology and WFSA
1954	Emeritus Professor, McGill
1954	*Mysterious Waters to Guard* published
	Canadian Anaesthetists' Society Journal started
1962	W. Bourne, H.R. Griffith and H.J. Shields first CAS gold medallists
1965	Died, Friday, 26th February, 1965, Montreal

Fontanus Publications

Fontanus (journal)

v.1 1988
v.2 1989
v.3 1990
v.4 1991
v.5 1992 Montreal 350th Anniversary Issue
v.6 1993 Redpath Issue
v.7 1994 Stephen Leacock Issue
v.8 1995 Women in the University Issue
v.9 1996 McGill 175th Anniversary Issue

Fontanus Monograph Series

I Adam Gacek, *Arabic Manuscripts in the Libraries of McGill University, Union Catalogue*, 1991
II Calvin Evans, *Sõren Kierkegaard Bibliographies: Remnants 1944-1980 and Multi-Media, 1925-1991*, 1993
III Barbara Lawson, *Collected Curios: Missionary Tales from the South Seas*, 1994
IV John Hobbins, *On the Edge of Greatness: The Diaries of John Humphrey, First Director of the United Nations Division of Human Rights, Vol. 1, 1948-1949*, 1994
V Max Dunbar, *Essays from a Life: Scotland, Canada, Greenland, Denmark*, 1995
VI Alberto Pérez-Gómez and Louise Pelletier, *Anamorphosis: An Annotated Bibliography with Special Reference to Architectural Representation*, 1995
VII Adam Gacek, *Arabic Lithographed Books in the Islamic Studies Library, McGill University, Descriptive Catalogue*, 1996
VIII Irena Žantovská Murray, *Sources in Iconography in the Blackader-Luaterman Library of Architecture and Art, McGill University, An Annotated Bibliography*, 1996
IX John Hobbins, *On the Edge of Greatness: The Diaries of John Humphrey, First Director of the United Nations Division of Human Rights, Vol. 2, 1950-1951*, 1996
X Joan C. Bevan and Maria A. Pacelli, *The Quintessential Canadian Anæsthetist: Wesley Bourne*, 1996

Orders may be placed at:

Marketing Department
McGill-Queen's University Press
3430 McTavish Street
Montreal QC
Canada H3A 1X9